Treat Your Own Knees

A self-help treatment plan to fully rehabilitate 26 common knee injuries and conditions

Brad Walker

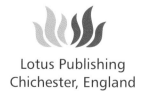

Lotus Publishing
Chichester, England

First published in 2011 by
Lotus Publishing
Apple Tree Cottage, Inlands Road, Nutbourne, Chichester, West Sussex, PO18 8RJ

All Drawings Amanda Williams
Text Design Wendy Craig
Cover Design Jim Wilkie
Printed and Bound in the UK by Scotprint

British Library Cataloguing-in-Publication Data
A CIP record for this book is available from the British Library
ISBN 978 1 905367 21 4

Contents

PART I—Knee Injury Diagnosis and Prevention

Introduction

The prominence of knee references in the English language – such as *knee-jerk reaction, the bee's knees, and knee deep* – should be enough of a hint as to the importance of the knee. At first sight, the knee may appear to be a simple joint, but it is actually quite complex. This complexity also makes the knee susceptible to many injuries, and the joint is often overlooked until something goes wrong. Healthy knees are generally happy knees, and keeping the knees healthy is much better than trying to rehabilitate them after an injury.

Function of the Knee

The knee serves several purposes and its main purpose is to allow forward and backward movement of the lower leg. Flexion and extension at the knee makes walking, jogging, running, jumping, and even sitting possible. It allows a change in the level of the body by means of the squatting motion. Flexion at the knee is also needed to decelerate when stopping after a sprint or landing from a jump.

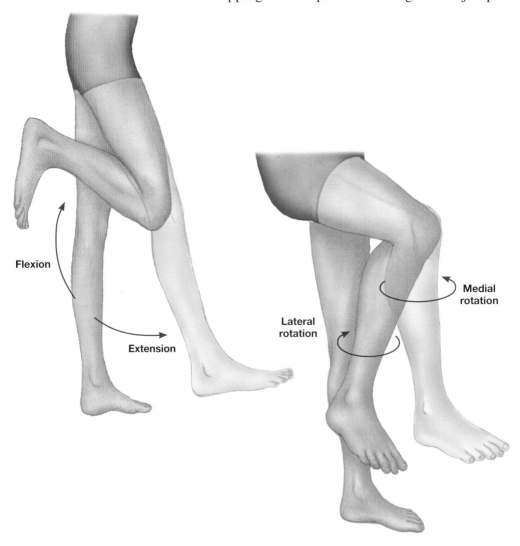

The knee also allows some rotational movement. This makes turning, direction changes, and other agility activities possible. The strong muscles and ligaments surrounding the knee keep it secure while allowing a minimal amount of rotation. The lubrication in the joint keeps it moving smoothly, even when slightly rotated.

The cartilage and space in the joint provide some shock-absorbing action as well, which reduces the stress placed on the spine. When walking, running, or jumping, an impact with the ground can send forces several times the bodyweight up through the skeletal system. The knee is the second stage in this shock-absorbing chain.

Importance of the Knee

The knee is the link between the foot and the core of the body. It is the joint that pulls it all together. The bones of the lower leg (*tibia* and *fibula*) are connected to the larger bone of the upper leg (*femur*) at the knee joint.

As stated above, the knee joint allows flexion and extension of the lower leg. This makes walking, running, and jumping possible. Bending the knee allows a person to reach items low to the ground and to sit down. Without the knee joint all movement in the lower extremities would have to come from the hips and ankles, leaving a very stiff action in the long bones of the leg.

The amount of stress placed on the spine during impact activities such as running would be several times greater without the shock-absorbing effect of the knee. The cartilage, bursa, and space in the knee are an essential part of the body's shock-absorbing system.

The knee is a key component in agility. The flexibility, strength, and structure of the knee allow it to be put through several different angles with different forces. The knee's complex nature allows these direction changes and mild rotation. This complex structure is also why it is more susceptible to injuries.

Anatomy of the Knee

Bones of the Knee

The knee joint connects the bones of the upper and lower legs. The distal head of the *femur* forms the top of the knee joint. The proximal head of the *tibia*, along with the *fibula*, forms the bottom of the knee joint. The *patella*, or kneecap, is a small sesamoid bone that rests over the anterior surface of the joint. These four bones come together to form the knee joint.

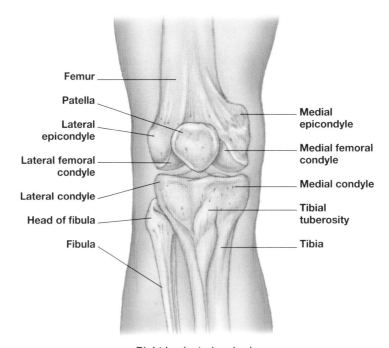

Femur

Patella

Lateral epicondyle

Lateral femoral condyle

Lateral condyle

Head of fibula

Fibula

Medial epicondyle

Medial femoral condyle

Medial condyle

Tibial tuberosity

Tibia

Right leg (anterior view)

Muscles of the Knee

The muscles around the knee joint are primarily responsible for both movement of the upper and lower leg, and stability of the knee joint. The major muscles at the front of the upper leg (or thigh) are the *sartorius* and the *quadriceps*, which include *rectus femoris*, *vastus medialis*, *vastus intermedius*, and *vastus lateralis*. The major muscles at the back of the upper leg are the *hamstrings*, which include *biceps femoris*, *semitendinosus*, and *semimembranosus*.

The major muscles on the inside of the upper leg are the *pectineus*, the *gracilis* and the *adductors*, which include *adductor brevis*, *adductor longus*, and *adductor magnus*. On the outside of the upper leg are the *tensor fasciae latae* and, to a lesser degree, the *gluteus* muscles, which include *gluteus maximus*, *gluteus medius*, and *gluteus minimus*.

The major muscles of the lower leg include *tibialis anterior* at the front of the lower leg, and the *gastrocnemius* and *soleus* at the back of the lower leg.

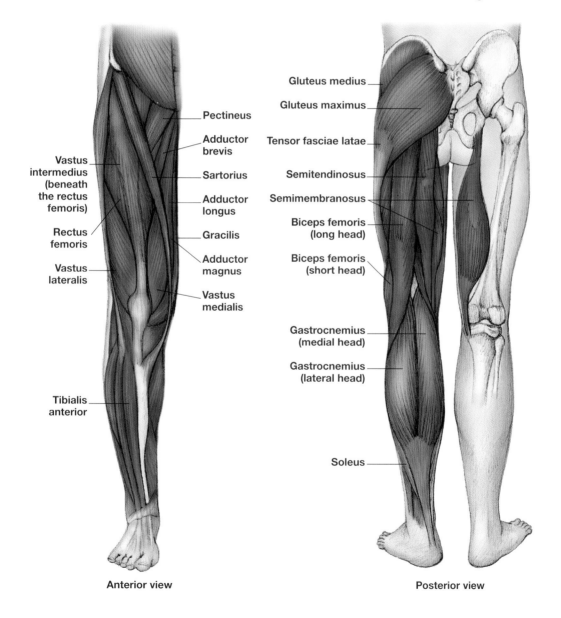

Anterior view   Posterior view

Ligaments of the Knee

The bones of a joint are held together by tough fibrous bands called *ligaments*. The knee is no different and has several ligaments. The knee is bordered on each side by ligaments that prevent lateral motion of the knee. The *lateral collateral ligament* (LCL) is on the outside of the knee and connects the femur to the head of the fibula. The *medial collateral ligament* (MCL) is on the inside of the knee and connects the femur to the tibia.

The *posterior cruciate ligament* (PCL) is located in the rear of the knee and connects the femur and the tibia from this location. It controls backward movement of the tibia. The *anterior cruciate ligament* (ACL) connects the tibia and femur in the center of the knee. It controls rotation and forward movement of the tibia. The LCL, MCL, PCL, and ACL are the four major ligaments of the knee.

There are also some minor ligaments that help add stability to the joint. The *transverse ligament* runs in front of the *lateral* and *medial menisci* and connects the two together. The *oblique* and *arcuate popliteal ligaments* round out the ligament structure.

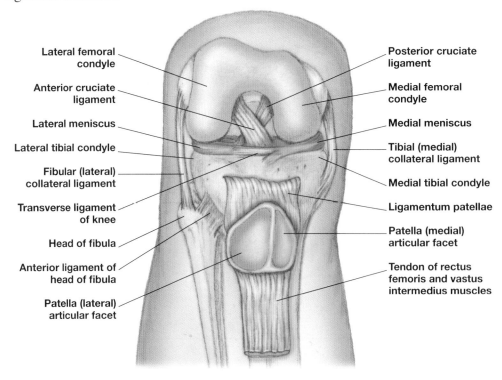

Lateral femoral condyle

Anterior cruciate ligament

Lateral meniscus

Lateral tibial condyle

Fibular (lateral) collateral ligament

Transverse ligament of knee

Head of fibula

Anterior ligament of head of fibula

Patella (lateral) articular facet

Posterior cruciate ligament

Medial femoral condyle

Medial meniscus

Tibial (medial) collateral ligament

Medial tibial condyle

Ligamentum patellae

Patella (medial) articular facet

Tendon of rectus femoris and vastus intermedius muscles

Right leg (anterior view)

Tendons of the Knee

The muscles are attached to the bones by strong fibrous tissues called *tendons* (as opposed to ligaments, which attach bone to bone). The largest tendon of the knee is the *quadriceps tendon*, which runs from the quadriceps muscles to the patella. It continues over and around the patella and becomes the *patellar tendon* below the bone to its attachment on the tibia.

The tendons of the hamstring complex run over the knee joint and connect to the tibia in the rear. The gastrocnemius tendon runs up from the gastrocnemius muscle, in the calf, to attach on the femur. The tendons of the tensor fasciae latae and the sartorius cross over the knee joint on opposite sides and attach to the lower leg.

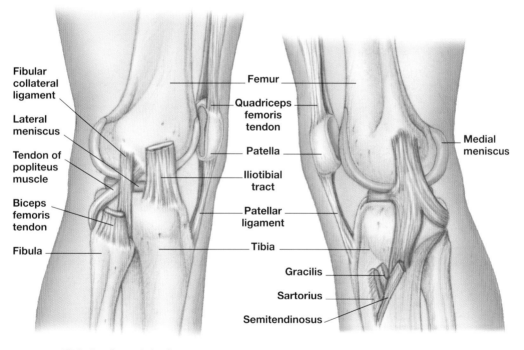

Right leg (lateral view)   Right leg (medial view)

Meniscus

Cartilage is found in joints on the end of bones to cushion and protect the bones. A *meniscus* is a crescent-shaped fibrocartilaginous structure. In humans it can be found in the knee among other joints. In the knee it is divided into two separate structures: the *lateral meniscus* and the *medial meniscus*. These menisci are attached to the head of the tibia.

The menisci serve to reduce friction between the tibia and the femur. They also disperse the body weight and act as shock absorbers. The menisci keep the joint moving smoothly and within the proper plane.

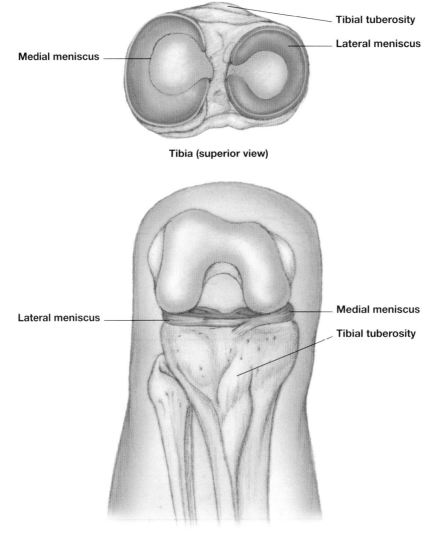

Tibial tuberosity

Lateral meniscus

Medial meniscus

Tibia (superior view)

Medial meniscus

Tibial tuberosity

Lateral meniscus

Knee in flexion (anterior view)

Synovium

The *synovium* is the membrane that lines the joint and secretes fluid for lubrication. The entire articular capsule is covered by the synovium. It is responsible for keeping the joint lubricated and protecting the cartilage.

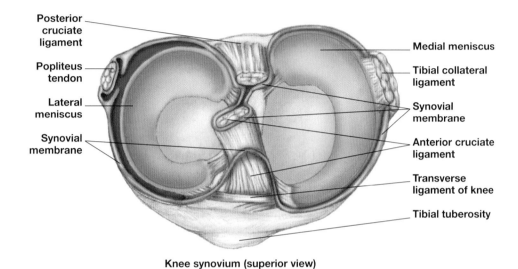

Posterior cruciate ligament

Popliteus tendon

Lateral meniscus

Synovial membrane

Medial meniscus

Tibial collateral ligament

Synovial membrane

Anterior cruciate ligament

Transverse ligament of knee

Tibial tuberosity

Knee synovium (superior view)

Bursae

Bursae are small sacs filled with synovial fluid. They cushion and protect the bones, tendons, and ligaments of most joints in the body. There are five major bursae in the anterior portion of the knee. The *suprapatellar bursa* rests on the head of the femur under the quadriceps tendon, allowing for smooth motion of the tendon over the bone. The *prepatellar bursa* rests atop the patella, between it and the skin. The *deep infrapatellar bursa* lies on top of the tibia, just under the patellar tendon. The *subcutaneous infrapatellar bursa* sits between the patellar tendon and the skin. Finally, the *pretibial bursa* is attached to the tibial tuberosity between the bone and the skin.

There are also four bursae on each side of the knee. Laterally, the *lateral gastrocnemius bursa* protects the articular capsule from the lateral head of the gastrocnemius. Medially, there is a mirror of that bursa, called the *medial gastrocnemius bursa*. The *fibular* and *fibulopopliteal bursae* rest between the LCL and the tendons of the muscles that run over them. On the medial side, the *pes anserine bursa* and the *bursa semimembranosa* do the same for the MCL and the tendons that cover it. The *subpopliteal bursa* protects the tendon of the popliteus from the lateral condyle of the femur. On the medial side, there is one more bursa that protects the tendon of the semimembranosus from the head of the tibia.

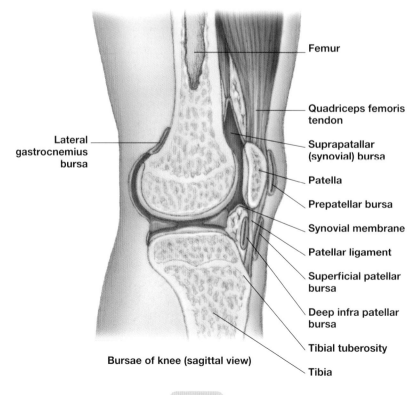

Bursae of knee (sagittal view)

Femur

Quadriceps femoris tendon

Suprapatallar (synovial) bursa

Patella

Prepatellar bursa

Synovial membrane

Patellar ligament

Superficial patellar bursa

Deep infra patellar bursa

Tibial tuberosity

Tibia

Lateral gastrocnemius bursa

Types of Knee Injury

Acute

Acute injuries are those that occur from a single traumatic event. They may be caused by excessive force placed on a joint, such as a blow to the area, forceful twisting, or force unevenly applied. For the knee, this could be caused by a blow to the lateral or medial side of the knee, forceful twisting of the knee with the foot in a fixed position, landing incorrectly, a forceful blow to the front of the knee, or even a force applied to the upper or lower leg. Tendons in the knee may be injured when the muscles have to act against a force beyond their strength level, especially when it is an explosive force or when the muscles are in a stretched position.

Common acute injuries of the knee include ligament sprains and tears (especially the MCL and ACL), meniscus tears, dislocations of the kneecap or knee joint, and tears to the patellar tendon. The quadriceps tendon may also be torn, and the LCL and PCL can be strained as well. The patella may be chipped or fractured, as may the head of the femur or tibia.

Acute injuries, if left untreated or if return to activity is too soon, can lead to chronic issues later. A properly treated and rehabilitated acute injury should not have lingering effects. Some injuries respond well to the normal course of R.I.C.E.R. (see below), while other, more severe injuries, may require surgery. In order to have a full return to activity with no lingering effects, it is important to follow the full treatment recommendations for the injury sustained.

Chronic

Chronic injuries, on the other hand, usually occur over time due to an improper wear, improper balance, or incorrect form issue. A chronic injury may be the result of an acute injury that was not allowed to heal properly. Muscle imbalances, poor form while doing activities involving the lower body, improper footwear, incorrect gait, or even continuous running on uneven or excessively hard surfaces may also lead to chronic knee injuries.

Although chronic knee injuries develop over time, this does not negate their severity. If allowed to continue they can cause severe pain and disability. The pain of chronic injuries may come and go at first, but over time this may develop into a constant pain that increases in severity with activity. Often, untreated chronic injuries lead to an involuntary cessation of activity due to the pain.

Chronic injuries of the knee include bursitis, patellar and quadriceps tendinitis, arthritis, and compartment syndrome (if wraps and braces are used incorrectly or acute injuries are not treated promptly). These injuries can often be avoided, or reversed, by correction of the underlying problem. Most chronic injuries develop as a result of the mistreatment of a correctable problem.

How Are Knee Injuries Classified?

As well as classifying a knee injury as *acute* or *chronic*, knee injuries are also classified according to their severity. Injuries are graded into one of three classifications: *mild*, *moderate*, and *severe*.

A *mild* knee injury will result in minimal pain and swelling. It will not adversely affect sporting performance, and the affected area is neither tender to touch nor deformed in any way. Examples of a mild knee injury include minor sprains, strains, and simple overuse injuries like tendinitis.

A *moderate* knee injury will result in some pain and swelling. It will have a limiting effect on sporting performance, and the affected area will be mildly tender to touch. Some discoloration at the injury site may also be present. Examples of a moderate knee injury include partial tearing of ligaments and other soft tissues.

A *severe* knee injury will result in increased pain and swelling. It will affect not only sporting performance, but also normal daily activities. The injury site is usually very tender to touch, and discoloration and deformity are common. Examples of a severe knee injury include dislocations, fractures, and ligament ruptures.

How Are Soft Tissue Injuries Classified?

The term *sprain* refers to an injury of the ligaments, as opposed to a *strain*, which refers to an injury of the muscles or tendons. Remember, ligaments attach bone to bone, whereas tendons attach muscle to bone.

Injuries to the ligaments, muscles, and tendons are usually graded into three categories: these types of injury are referred to as *Grade 1*, *Grade 2*, and *Grade 3* sprains and strains.

A *Grade 1* sprain/strain is the least severe. It is the result of some minor stretching of the ligaments, muscles, or tendons and is accompanied by mild pain, some swelling, and joint stiffness. There is usually very little loss of joint stability as a result of a Grade 1 sprain/strain.

A *Grade 2* sprain/strain is the result of both stretching and some tearing of the ligaments, muscles, or tendons. There is increased swelling and pain associated with a Grade 2 sprain/strain, and a moderate loss of stability around the knee joint.

A *Grade 3* sprain/strain is the most severe of the three. It is the result of a complete tear or rupture of one or more of the ligaments, muscles, and tendons. A Grade 3 sprain/strain will result in massive swelling, severe pain, and gross instability of the knee joint.

Knee Injury Prevention

Risk Factors

There are many variables that may predispose someone to knee injuries. Most of these can be corrected or reversed, and prevention is most definitely a much better option than repair, especially since one of the risk factors for knee injuries is *previous injury*. Having injured the knee on a prior occasion makes it more susceptible to a recurrence of that (or another) injury. Preventing injuries has therefore a twofold effect in that respect.

Lack of conditioning is another risk factor for knee injury. If the muscles, ligaments, and tendons around the knee are not properly conditioned for the stresses placed on them, injury may result. This can be either a chronic overuse injury or an acute traumatic injury. Stresses that go beyond the current conditioning level of the muscles and joint can cause injury.

Muscle imbalances, like poor conditioning, can quickly lead to both chronic and acute injuries to the knee. They are just as preventable too. When an imbalance occurs, the stronger muscle (or the more flexible muscle) may overpower the weaker ones and cause the joint to move in an improper line or at awkward angles. This can cause irregular stress on the joint and the ligaments that hold it together. It also stresses the cartilage and bursae in the knee, which can lead to acute tears or chronic wear issues.

Overuse and *incorrect use* are other common causes of knee injury. Overuse injuries may result from increasing the workload too quickly or from chronic overuse. Incorrect use generally relates to form issues. Performing movements incorrectly or with improper form can lead to acute injury to the joint. Continued incorrect form can lead to chronic overuse injury.

Being overweight also places excessive stress on the knee joint. Every step, even while walking, results in forces several times the bodyweight being sent through the knee joint. Even heavily muscled athletes may experience injury to the knee joint due to the extra weight and impact. However, individuals who are overweight and have poor conditioning are much more likely to experience chronic and acute knee injuries.

Reversing these risk factors will help prevent knee injuries before they occur. All of these factors can be addressed with proper training. Conditioning the body, especially the muscles of the legs, to the activities that are expected of it will help reduce the stress on the knee joint. Reducing muscle imbalances and correcting form issues will also reduce stress and chronic wear on the joint. Reducing overall bodyweight will lower the impact on the joint as well.

Strength

Strong muscles around the knee joint provide support. These muscles must be strong enough to absorb the shock of the forces they experience each time the foot hits the ground. They must be strong enough to support the knee, even when forces act on it from various angles.

Strengthening the muscles around the knee (the quadriceps, hamstrings, adductors, abductors, gastrocnemius, soleus, and tibialis anterior) will provide the necessary support. The muscles, through the network of tendons that cross the joint, take a large amount of the stress that is applied to the joint. Strong muscles can absorb more stress each time. These muscles also provide support against hyperflexion and hyperextension.

Flexibility

As with strength, flexibility applies to the muscles and tendons around the knee joint. Tight muscles put excessive pressure on the joint, even during rest. When muscles are tight they may pull the joints at unnatural angles, which may also cause muscle imbalances.

Tight muscles are more susceptible to strains, and these strains may lead to additional imbalances and continued inflexibility. Flexible muscles not only allow a wider range of motion, but also have a greater degree of strength at each end of that range. Flexible muscles are stronger muscles.

Balance

The knees are key to overall balance of the body. Good muscle balance around the knee will ensure adequate support when the knee is placed under normal stress. Muscle imbalances can quickly lead to injury due to irregular stress placed on the knee. Chronic imbalances can cause damage to the ligaments and cartilage in the knee, as well as putting extra pressure on the bursae.

Balance applies to an overall muscular balance in the body, as well. Poor overall balance can lead to knee injuries too. Weak muscles in the core can cause problems during change of direction and explosive movements. The muscles surrounding the knee have to work harder to maintain balance and total body support when the muscles of the core are weak.

Knee health relies on good balance in the muscles around the knee, as well as the overall balance of muscles in the body, especially the core. Poor body balance can easily put too much stress on the knee by allowing the knee to be placed under excessive stress in awkward positions. Proper muscle balance reduces those stresses and provides the proper support.

Proprioception

When a soft tissue injury occurs to the knee, there is always a certain amount of damage to the nerves around the injured area. This, of course, leads to a lack of control of the muscles and tendons, and can also affect the stability of the joint structure.

Without this information the muscles, tendons and ligaments around the knee are constantly second-guessing the position of the joint and limbs. This lack of awareness about the position of the joint and limbs (*proprioception*) can lead to a re-occurrence of the same injury long after it was thought to be completely healed.

Proprioceptive exercises are important to help retrain the damaged nerves around the injured knee. Start with simple balancing exercises such as walking along a straight line or balancing on a beam. Progress to one-leg exercises, for example balancing on one foot, and then perform the same exercises with your eyes closed. When comfortable with the above activities, try some of the more advanced exercises using wobble or rocker boards, Swiss balls, stability cushions, and foam rollers.

Braces and Support

After an injury, or while working through imbalances, braces and other supports may help to provide the support needed to keep the knee healthy. Commercial braces, or taping or wrapping the knee, may provide the appropriate support during athletic activities. When the body cannot provide its own support, these braces may provide an artificial support to supplement the body's own ability.

During activities where the knee may be placed under excessive stress, knee supports may be needed to augment the body's own support. After an injury the muscles, tendons or ligaments may not be as strong as they should be, so braces or supports provide the additional protection needed until the injury heals and is properly rehabilitated.

There are many commercially available braces ranging from cloth-like material braces to those with titanium support rods or made of molded fiberglass or Kevlar material. These braces may be available in standard sizes or molded to fit a particular user.

Taping or wrapping may be done to provide additional support as well. Care must be used when taping or wrapping to ensure that the tape or wrap does not create unusual pull or excessive strain on the joint. Ensuring proper support for the injured or weak area must also be taken into consideration. Whenever possible the tape or wrap should be applied by a sports medicine professional, or at least proper training should be undertaken before self-taping.

Diagnosis and Tests

Diagnosing a knee injury requires looking at the signs and symptoms, and often an x-ray or MRI. The onset of pain, either instant or over time, may also indicate the type of injury. It is important to take into consideration all of the signs and symptoms when diagnosing a knee injury. Many injuries present similar symptoms.

Acute injuries, as stated above, occur very quickly; chronic injuries generally occur over time. Pain may be sharp, dull, burning, or a combination. It may come and go or it may be constant. It may occur only during activity or it may continue even during rest. These pain indicators will help to diagnose the problem, and often determine the underlying cause of the injury as well.

Strains and sprains usually cause weakness and guarding of the injury, and pain is generally located at the injury site. Some swelling will generally occur over the injury site as well. Fractures and dislocations will result in swelling over that region and often inability to bear weight, usually accompanied by severe pain. Bursitis and meniscus tears are usually accompanied by dull pain and pressure in the knee. A clicking or popping may be felt in the knee during movement and the pain is worse with movement and decreases during rest.

Most knee injuries require a sports medicine professional or physician for accurate diagnosis. Minor injuries like strains and minor sprains can often be diagnosed by the athlete, but more severe injuries should be attended to by a physician. X-rays or MRIs may be needed to accurately diagnose the injury. A sports medicine specialist's experience may also be helpful in making a diagnosis from the signs and symptoms presented.

Knee Injury Examinations and Tests

A number of specialized examinations and tests can be used to help diagnose the type of knee injury sustained. However, before any formal tests are conducted, the first course of action should be a simple visual inspection of the injured knee, by comparing it to the uninjured knee, and an informal request for information such as: *Where does it hurt? How did the injury occur?*

Next, the examiner should use simple movement and palpation tests to further identify the exact location of any pain. The examiner should also look for symptoms such as knee joint locking, which is an indication of damage to the cartilage and/or meniscus, and knee joint instability, which is an indication of damage to the ligaments of the knee.

The information gathered during this pre-test procedure should help the examiner decide on the type of tests required for a further, and more complete, diagnosis. The following are a number of specialized tests to help further diagnose the type of injury sustained.

Lachman Test: *Used to help diagnose an ACL injury.*
The patient lies flat while the examiner bends the knee to about 30 degrees. The examiner then stabilizes the femur and pulls the top of the tibia upward (anteriorly). Excessive upward movement indicates damage to the ACL.

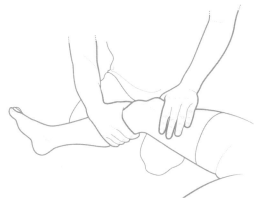

Posterolateral Lachman Test: *Used to help diagnose an injury to the structures of the posterolateral corner of the knee (LCL, popliteus tendon, popliteofibular ligament).*
The patient lies face up while the examiner bends the knee to about 30 degrees. The examiner then stabilizes the femur and pushes the top of the tibia downward (posteriorly), with the leg in an externally rotated position. Excessive downward movement indicates damage to the posterolateral structures.

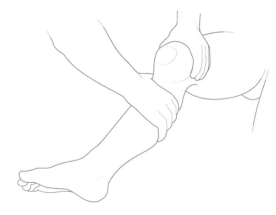

Anterior Drawer Test: *Used to help diagnose an ACL injury.*
The patient lies face up while the examiner bends the knee to about 90 degrees. The examiner pulls the top of the tibia forward. Excessive forward movement indicates damage to the ACL.

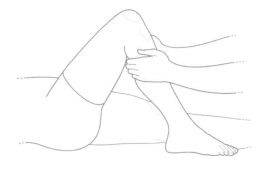

Posterior Drawer Test: *Used to help diagnose a PCL injury.*
The patient lies face up while the examiner bends the knee to about 90 degrees. The examiner pushes the top of the tibia rearward. Excessive rearward movement indicates damage to the PCL.

Sag Test: *Used to help diagnose a PCL injury.*
The patient lies face up while the examiner bends both the hip and the knee to 90 degrees. In this position the top of the tibia will sag downward if the PCL is damaged. Excessive downward movement, compared to the healthy side, indicates damage to the PCL.

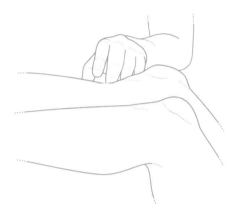

Varus Instability Test: *Used to help diagnose an LCL injury.*
The patient lies face up while the examiner bends the knee to about 30 degrees. While holding the lower leg the examiner moves the tibia medially. Excessive medial movement, along with opening of the lateral side of the knee, indicates damage to the LCL.

Valgus Instability Test: *Used to help diagnose an MCL injury.*
The patient lies face up while the examiner bends the knee to about 30 degrees. While holding the lower leg the examiner moves the tibia laterally. Excessive lateral movement, along with opening of the medial side of the knee, indicates damage to the MCL.

Dial Test: *Used to help diagnose an injury to the structures of the posterolateral corner of the knee (LCL, popliteus tendon, popliteofibular ligament).*
The patient lies face down while the examiner bends both knees to about 30 degrees. The examiner rotates both feet outward. Excessive outward rotation, compared to the healthy side, indicates damage to the posterolateral structures.

Recurvatum Test: *Used to help diagnose an injury to the posterolateral ligament.*
The patient lies face up while the examiner lifts both feet about 10cm. Excessive passive hyperextension (downward movement) of the injured knee, compared to the healthy side, indicates damage to the posterolateral ligament.

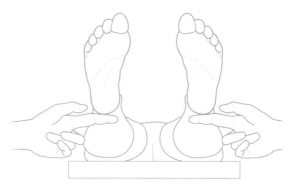

McMurray's Test: *Used to help diagnose a meniscus injury.*
The patient lies face up while the examiner flexes and extends the knee through its full range of motion. To test the medial meniscus the examiner feels for a clicking at the medial joint line while the tibia is in external rotation. To test the lateral meniscus the examiner feels for a clicking at the lateral joint line while the tibia is in internal rotation.

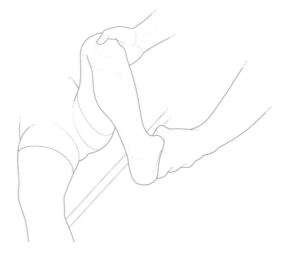

Ege's Test: *Used to help diagnose a meniscus injury.*
The patient stands with the feet about 25cm apart and performs a squat. Pain or a click is felt as the knee flexes past 90 degrees. To test the medial meniscus, the patient turns the feet outward, whereas turning the feet inward will test the lateral meniscus.

Patellar Grind Test: *Used to help diagnose a kneecap (or patellar) injury.*
The examiner feels for abnormal grinding by placing pressure on the kneecap and moving the knee joint through a full range of motion.

Patellar Apprehension Test: *Used to help diagnose kneecap instability.*
The patient lies face up with the knee flexed to about 30 degrees. The examiner feels for pain and excessive movement while placing lateral pressure on the kneecap.

Knee Surgery

Severe knee injuries may require surgery to correct and treat. Major ligament tears, meniscus tears, bursitis that does not respond to regular treatment, and some fractures and dislocations may all require surgery to repair. Surgery does increase the overall recovery time, but may be the only option to completely repair the joint.

Any injury that does not respond to normal treatment may require surgical repair, but surgery should not be taken lightly. Additional scarring and prolonged recovery can be an issue. In some cases, however, surgery is the only option.

There are different types of surgery that may be required for knee injuries. Three of the possible interventions that may be used are discussed below.

Closed Reduction
Although not a traditional "surgical" intervention, the closed reduction is considered surgery because it often requires some form of sedation. A closed reduction is used for dislocations. The bones are placed back in line using manual manipulation without requiring any incision or opening of the joint.

Adequate analgesia must be used to dull the pain senses in the area, and the bones are then moved to position them back in proper alignment. This method is much less invasive and reduces overall recovery time. However, it does not correct ligament or tendon tears. This method can also be used when the fractured ends of a bone are misaligned and need to be placed back in line before casting.

Closed reduction is often used with dislocations of the patella or when the knee joint becomes dislocated without major ligament tears requiring surgical repair. Closed reduction is usually followed by a period of time in a full leg brace to allow the soft tissue of the knee to heal. This may also be accompanied by a period of non-weight bearing on the affected leg.

Due to the extensive soft tissue involvement with a dislocation, recovery time is generally a little longer than for an isolated sprain. During, and immediately following, the immobilization phase a period of rehabilitation will be required to regain strength and range of motion in the joint.

Arthroscopic

Arthroscopic surgery has greatly reduced the recovery time for many knee injuries. The use of arthroscopy reduces the overall trauma on the joint because it does not require a large opening in the joint to correct the problem. This form of surgery is often used to repair meniscus tears and minor ligament issues.

Arthroscopic surgery can usually be done under local anesthetic and as an outpatient procedure. Weight bearing may resume to the extent that it can be tolerated, often within the first few days. Recovery usually takes only a few weeks, although ligament repairs generally take slightly longer to completely heal than meniscus repairs.

The surgery is performed using one or two small tools inserted through very small incisions on each side of the knee, along with a scope to transmit images of the area inside the joint to the surgeon. These small incisions heal much quicker than larger ones from more invasive procedures. The small amount of air and fluid pushed into the joint during arthroscopy is quickly absorbed by the body, and the swelling and inflammation subside much quicker also.

Arthroscopic surgery requires a short recovery period, and since weight bearing is resumed shortly after, rehabilitation can begin almost immediately following the surgery. Range of motion may be an issue at first, but with gentle work it will return. Strength recovery should be quick after arthroscopy as well.

Open

Major knee injuries, especially those requiring reconstruction of ligaments, menisci or the joint itself, often call for open surgery. This procedure involves an incision into the joint to facilitate repair of the joint. It is much more invasive than the other two procedures, and therefore usually requires a longer recovery period.

Open surgery is often used for injuries such as major ACL tears, major trauma to multiple ligaments, meniscus or total knee replacement, and other major knee injuries that are too complex for arthroscopic surgery or require surgical reattachment. This is a "hands-on" approach to surgery. The surgeon can get right into the joint and make the necessary repairs, then close it back up. Open surgery normally requires a general anesthetic or a spinal block.

The major trauma involved in this type of surgery will usually require knee immobilization and no (or reduced) weight bearing on the affected leg. This means a period of rehabilitation to return to a normal range of motion and to regain strength. Rehabilitation can generally begin even before the brace is removed, as long as care is taken not to aggravate the injury.

Open, invasive surgery should be a last resort. It causes additional damage to the joint, beyond the initial injury, that requires additional recovery time. This also opens the door for post-surgical infection and, in the long term, additional arthritis in the joint.

PART II—Knee Injury Management and Rehabilitation

This part is divided into two distinct sections:

1. The theory behind injury rehabilitation, which is designed to provide an overview of the stages the body goes through during the healing process.

2. A detailed set of practical exercises, stretches, and drills that can be used to fully rehabilitate the injured knee.

Theory

Please note: while the following information is specifically applicable to acute injuries of the knee, it is just as valid (and can be easily adapted) for chronic injuries.

First Aid: The First Three Minutes

Before moving on to the specifics of knee injury treatment, it is important to take a minute to discuss the period immediately following a knee injury, or any sports injury for that matter.

The first three minutes after an injury occurs are crucial. It is the time when an initial assessment of the injury is made and appropriate steps are taken to minimize trauma and prevent further damage. This is the first priority when treating any sports injury.

Before treating any injury, whether to yourself or someone else, first STOP and take account of what has occurred. Consider the following: *Is the area safe from other dangers? Is there a threat to life? Is the injury serious enough to seek emergency help?* Then, using the word STOP as an acronym . . .

S: (stop) Stop the injured athlete from moving. Consider stopping the sport or game if necessary.

T: (talk) Ask questions such as: *What happened? How did it happen? What did it feel like? Where does it hurt? Have you injured this before?*

O: (observe) Look and feel for things like swelling, bruising, deformity, and tenderness.

P: (prevent) Remember, do no further damage. Prevent further injury.

Now make an assessment of the severity of the injury:

1. Is it a *mild* injury? Is it a bump or bruise that does not impair the athlete's physical performance? If so, play on. Provide a few words of encouragement, monitor the injury, and apply the treatment procedures described in the next section just to be on the safe side.

2. Is it a *moderate* injury? Is it a sprain, strain, or severe bruise that impairs the athlete's ability to play on? If so, get the player off the field and apply the treatment procedures described in the next section as soon as possible.

3. Is it a *severe* injury? Does the injury affect the head, neck, face, or spinal cord? Does it involve shock, excessive bleeding, or bone fractures and breaks? The treatment of these types of injury goes way beyond the relatively simple soft tissue injury treatment. *Seek professional help immediately.*

Once a few moments have been taken to make sure the injury is not life threatening, it is then time to start treating the injury. The sooner treatment is started, the greater chance the injured athlete will have of a full and complete recovery.

Treatment: The Next Three Days

Without a doubt, the most effective initial treatment for soft tissue injuries is the R.I.C.E.R. regimen. This involves the application of **R**est, **I**ce, **C**ompression, and **E**levation, and obtaining a **R**eferral for diagnosis and appropriate medical treatment.

Where the R.I.C.E.R. regimen has been used immediately after the occurrence of an injury, it has been shown to significantly reduce recovery time. R.I.C.E.R. forms the first, and perhaps the most important, stage of injury rehabilitation, providing the early base for the complete recovery from injury.

When a soft tissue injury occurs there is a large amount of uncontrolled bleeding around the injury site. The excessive bleeding causes swelling that puts pressure on nerve endings and results in increased pain. It is exactly this process of bleeding, swelling, and pain that the R.I.C.E.R. regimen will help to alleviate. The procedure will also limit tissue damage and aid the healing process.

Rest: It is important that the injured knee be kept as still as possible. If necessary support the entire leg with a splint or brace. This will help to slow blood flow to the injured area and prevent any further damage.

Ice: This is by far the most important part! The application of ice will have the greatest effect on reducing bleeding, swelling, and pain. Apply ice as soon as possible after the injury has occurred.

How do you apply ice? Crushed ice in a plastic bag is usually best. However, blocks of ice, commercial cold packs, and bags of frozen peas will all do fine. Even cold water from a tap is better than nothing at all.

When using ice, be careful not to apply it directly to the skin. This can cause *ice burns* and further skin damage. Wrapping the ice in a damp towel generally provides the best protection for the skin.

How long? How often? This is the point where few people agree. The following are some figures to use as a rough guide, and then some advice from personal experience will be offered. The most common recommendation is to apply ice for 20 minutes every 2 hours for the first 48 to 72 hours.

These figures are a good starting point, but remember, they are only a guide. A number of precautions must be taken into account, including:
• Some people are more sensitive to cold than others
• Children and elderly people have a lower tolerance to ice and cold
• People with circulatory problems are also more sensitive to ice

The safest recommendation is that people use their own judgment when applying ice to the injured area. For some people, 20 minutes will be way too long. For others, especially well-conditioned athletes, the ice can be left on for a lot longer.

The individual should make the decision as to how long the ice stays on. People should apply ice for as long as is comfortable. Obviously, there will be a slight discomfort from the cold, but as soon as pain or excessive discomfort is experienced, it is time to remove the ice. It is much better to apply ice for 3 to 5 minutes, a couple of times an hour, than not at all.

Compression: Compression actually achieves two things. Firstly, it helps to reduce both the bleeding and the swelling around the injured area; and secondly, it provides support for the injured knee. Simply use a wide, firm, elastic compression bandage to cover the injured part, being sure to bandage both above and below the injured knee.

Elevation: If possible, have the individual lie down and raise the injured leg above the level of the heart. This will further help to reduce the bleeding and swelling.

Referral: If the injury is severe enough, it is important that the injured person consult a professional physical therapist or a qualified sports doctor for an accurate diagnosis of the injury. With an accurate diagnosis, the individual can then move on to a specific rehabilitation program to further reduce recovery time.

A Word of Warning!
Before moving on, there are a few things that must be avoided during the first 48 to 72 hours after an injury. Be sure to avoid any form of heat at the injury site. This includes heat lamps, heat creams, spas, Jacuzzis, and saunas. Avoid all movement and massage of the injured area. Also avoid alcohol. All these things will increase the bleeding, swelling, and pain of your injury.

Medication
Non-steroidal anti-inflammatory drugs (NSAIDs) are very common in the treatment of acute and chronic injuries. They help reduce the inflammation in the injured joint, allowing for more rapid healing. They also have some pain-relieving effects.

Over-the-counter and prescription pain medications are also common in injury treatment. Reducing pain in the injured joint allows the body to heal quicker. These medications permit movement as needed for rehabilitation activities. However, they are not meant to mask the pain so that a person can return to activity before the injury has healed.

Muscle relaxants may be used for muscle strains, and even sprains, when the muscles are tight or experiencing spasms. These medications are intended to reduce the stress on the joint from the muscles, allowing the tendons or ligaments to heal.

Initial Rehabilitation: The Next Three Weeks
It is very important that a full diagnosis of the injury is completed first, before any rehabilitation is started. This is because some treatment strategies, such as massage, are not appropriate for injuries that result in damage to some of the structures of the knee, like the meniscus and bursa.

When soft tissues, such as muscles, tendons and ligaments, are torn or damaged, it would be reasonable to expect that the body would repair that damage with new muscle, or ligament if a ligament is damaged, and so on. In reality, this does not happen. The tear, or damage, is repaired with *scar tissue*.

When the R.I.C.E.R. regimen is used immediately after a soft tissue injury occurs, the formation of scar tissue will be limited. However, some scar tissue will still be present.

This might not sound like a big deal, but for anyone who has ever suffered a soft tissue injury, they will know how annoying it is to keep re-injuring that same old injury, over and over again. Untreated scar tissue is a major cause of re-injury, usually months after it was thought that the injury had fully healed.

Scar tissue is made from a tough, inflexible fibrous material called *collagen*. This fibrous material binds itself to the damaged soft tissue fibers in an effort to draw the damaged fibers back together. What results is a bulky mass of fibrous scar tissue completely surrounding the injury site. In some cases it is even possible to see and feel this bulky mass under the skin.

When scar tissue forms around an injury site, it is never as strong as the tissue it replaces. It also has a tendency to contract and deform the surrounding tissues, so not only is the strength of the tissue diminished, but flexibility of the tissue is also compromised.

So what does this mean? Firstly, it means a shortening of the soft tissues, resulting in a loss of flexibility. Secondly, it means a weak spot has formed within the soft tissues, which could easily lead to further damage or re-injury. Lastly, the formation of scar tissue will result in a loss of strength and power. For a muscle to attain full power it must be fully stretched before contraction. Both the shortening effect and the weakening of the tissues mean that a full stretch and optimum contraction is not possible.

Getting Rid of the Scar Tissue
To minimize and re-align the unwanted scar tissue, two vital treatments need to be initiated.

The first is commonly used by physical therapists (or physiotherapists) and primarily involves increasing the blood supply to the injured area. The aim is to increase the amount of oxygen and nutrients to the damaged tissues. Physical therapists accomplish this aim by using a number of activities to stimulate the injured area. The most common methods used are ultrasound and heat.

Ultrasound, or TENS (transcutaneous electrical nerve stimulation), simply uses a light electrical pulse to stimulate the affected area. Heat, in the form of a ray lamp or hot water bottle, is very effective in stimulating blood flow to the damaged tissues.

Another treatment that may be used to minimize and re-align the unwanted scar tissue is deep tissue sports massage. While ultrasound and heat will help the injured area, they will not re-align the scar tissue – only massage will do that.

Either find someone who can massage the muscles around the knee, or, if possible, massage the damaged tissues yourself. Doing it yourself has the advantage of knowing just how hard and how deep you need to massage.

For improved soft tissue recovery a special massage ointment called *arnica* is recommended. This special ointment is extremely effective in treating soft tissue injuries such as sprains, strains, and tears.

Also, be sure to drink plenty of fluid during the injury rehabilitation process. The extra fluid will help to flush a lot of the waste products from the body.

A Word of Warning!
Please remember that massage and some other rehabilitation strategies are not appropriate for all types of knee injury. Please refer to the injury list in part III for specific rehabilitation strategies for each type of injury.

Active Rehabilitation
As part of the rehabilitation phase the injured athlete will be required to do exercises and activities that will help to speed up the recovery process. Some people refer to this phase of the recovery process as the *active rehabilitation phase*, because during this phase the athlete or individual is responsible for the rehabilitation process.

The aim of this phase of the recovery will be to regain all the fitness components that were lost during the injury process. Regaining flexibility, strength, power, muscular endurance, balance, and co-ordination will be the primary focus.

Without this phase of the rehabilitation process, there is no hope of completely and permanently making a full recovery from your injury. A quote from *Sporting*

Injuries by Peter Dornan and Richard Dunn (1987) will help to reinforce the value of active rehabilitation:

> *The injury symptoms will permanently disappear only after the patient has undergone a very specific exercise program, deliberately designed to stretch and strengthen and regain all parameters of fitness of the damaged structure or structures. Further, it is suggested that when a specific stretching program is followed, thus more permanently reorganizing the scar fibres and allowing the circulation to become normal, the painful symptoms will disappear permanently.*

The first point to make clear is how important it is to keep active. Often, the advice from doctors and similar medical personnel will simply be to rest. This can be one of the worst things an injured person can do. Without some form of activity the injured area will not receive the blood flow it requires for recovery. An active circulation will provide both the oxygen and the nutrients needed for the injury to heal.

Any form of gentle activity not only promotes blood circulation, but also activates the lymphatic system. The lymphatic system is vital in clearing the body of toxins and waste products that accumulate in the body following a serious injury. Activity is the only way to activate the lymphatic system.

Dornan and Dunn also support this approach:

> *One does not need to wait for full anatomical healing before starting to retrain the muscle. The retraining can be started, gradually at first, during the healing period. This same principle applies also to ligamentous and tendon injuries.*

A Word of Warning!

Never do any activity that hurts the injured area or causes pain. Of course, some discomfort may be felt, but never push the injured knee to the point where pain is experienced. The recovery process is a long journey. Do not take a step backward by over-exerting the injured knee. Be very careful with any activity. Pain is the warning sign – do not ignore it.

Long-term Rehabilitation: Regaining Lost Fitness Components

Now is the time to work on regaining the fitness components that were lost as a result of the injury. The main areas that need to be worked on are range of motion, flexibility, strength, and co-ordination.

Depending on the background of the athlete, and the type of sport that the athlete was engaged in, these elements should be the first priority. As the athlete begins to regain strength, flexibility, and co-ordination, they can then start to work on the more specific areas of their chosen sport.

1. Range of Motion

Regaining a full range of motion is the first priority in this phase of the rehabilitation process. A full range of motion is extremely important, as it lays the foundation for more intense and challenging exercises later in the active rehabilitation process.

While working through the initial stages of recovery, the injury will begin to heal and the athlete can start to introduce some very gentle movement-based exercises. First, begin bending and straightening the injured leg; then, as this becomes more comfortable, start to incorporate rotation exercises. Turn the injured area from side to side, and rotate clockwise and anti-clockwise.

Dornan and Dunn emphasize:

> *It is important that gentle stretching exercises be initiated early if normal flexibility is to be regained. For example, by actively stretching bruises of the thigh to their fullest pain-free extent, adhesion formation was limited and the thigh muscles were able to return to the pre-injury range of motion.*

When these range of motion exercises can be performed relatively pain free, it is time to move on to the next phase of the active rehabilitation process.

2. Stretch and Strengthen

At this point increased intensity is added to the range of motion exercises. The aim is to gradually re-introduce some flexibility and strength into the injured structures around the knee.

When attempting to increase the flexibility and strength of the injured area, be sure to approach this in a gradual, systematic way by lightly overloading the injured knee. Be careful not to overdo this type of training – patience is required.

The use of machine weights can be very effective for improving the strength of the injured area, because they provide a certain amount of stability to the joints and muscles as the athlete performs the rehabilitation exercises.

Another effective and relatively safe way to start is with *isometric exercises*. These are exercises where the injured knee does not move, yet force is applied and the muscles of the injured leg are contracted. To illustrate this, sit in a chair while facing a wall and then place the ball of your foot against the wall. In this position you can push against the wall with your foot and at the same time keep your knee joint from moving. The muscles contract but the knee joint does not move. This is an isometric exercise.

It is also important at this stage to introduce some gentle stretching exercises. These will help to further increase the range of motion and prepare the injury for more strenuous activity to come.

Remember, while working on increasing the flexibility of the injured area, it is also important to increase the flexibility of the muscle groups *around* the injured area. In the case of an injured knee, these would include the calf muscles, the anterior muscles of the shin, the quadriceps muscles, the hamstring muscles, and even the muscles of the lower back and hips.

3. Balance and Proprioception
This phase of the rehabilitation process is often overlooked and is another reason why old injuries keep re-occurring. When a soft tissue injury happens, there is always a certain amount of damage to the nerves around the injured area. This, of course, leads to a lack of control of the muscles and tendons, and can also affect the stability of joint structures.

Without this information the muscles, tendons, and ligaments are constantly second-guessing the position of the joints and limbs around the injured area. This lack of awareness about the position of the limbs (*proprioception*) can lead to a re-occurrence of the same injury long after it was thought to be completely healed.

When improved flexibility and strength have returned to the injured knee it is time to incorporate some balancing drills and exercises. Balancing exercises are important to help retrain the damaged nerves around the injured knee. Start with simple balancing exercises, such as walking along a straight line or balancing on a beam; progress to one-leg exercises, for example balancing on one foot; and then perform the same exercises with closed eyes. When comfortable with the above activities, try some of the more advanced exercises using wobble or rocker boards, Swiss balls, stability cushions, and foam rollers.

4. Final Preparation

This last part of the rehabilitation process will aim to return the knee joint to a pre-injury state. By the end of this process the injured knee should be as strong as, if not stronger than, it was before the injury occurred.

This is the time to incorporate some dynamic or explosive exercises to really strengthen up the injured area and improve proprioception. Start by working through all the exercises done during the previous stages of recovery, but with more intensity. For example, if you were using light isometric exercises to help strengthen the quadriceps muscles, start to apply more force or use some weighted exercises.

Next, gradually introduce some more intense exercises. Exercises that relate specifically to the athlete's chosen sport are a good place to start. Activities like skill drills and training exercises are a great way to gauge the fitness level and strength of the injured knee.

To put the finishing touches to the recovery, incorporate simple plyometric drills. *Plyometric exercises* are explosive exercises that both lengthen and contract a muscle at the same time. These are called *eccentric muscle contractions* and involve activities such as jumping, hopping, skipping, and bounding.

These activities are quite intense, so remember to start off easy and gradually apply more and more force. Do not get too excited and overdo it – patience and common sense are required.

Conditioning: The Next Three to Six Months

Where the above treatment procedures have been diligently applied, most soft tissue injuries of the knee will have completely healed. However, even though the initial injury may have healed and the individual is able to return to normal activities, it is important to continue further strength and conditioning exercises to prevent a repeat of the initial injury.

The goal of the next three to six months is to identify the underlying causes, or reasons why the injury occurred in the first place, and then, once these have been identified, employ conditioning exercises or training aids that will help to prevent a re-occurrence of the initial injury.

To accomplish this phase effectively, it is important to understand why sports injuries occur. Broadly speaking there are three main causes. The first is *accident*, the second is *overload*, and the third is *biomechanical error*.

Accidents: Accidents include things such as stepping into a pothole and spraining a knee, tripping over and falling onto the knee, and being struck by sporting equipment. While there is little that can be done to prevent some accidents, it is important to minimize these as much as possible. A little bit of common sense, and diligently employing some of the prevention techniques discussed earlier, will help to minimize injuries caused by accidents.

Overload: Overload is common with most sports and occurs when the structures within the body become fatigued and overworked. The structures then lose their ability to adequately perform their required task, which results in excessive strain (or overload) on other parts of the body.

For example, when the tensor fasciae latae muscle and iliotibial band, located in the thigh, become fatigued and overloaded, they lose their ability to adequately stabilize the entire leg. This in turn places stress on the knee joint, which results in pain and damage to the structures that make up the joint.

Most overload symptoms can be quickly reversed with adequate rest. However, there are a number of things that will contribute to overload and should be avoided. They include:
• Exercising on hard surfaces, such as concrete
• Exercising on uneven ground
• Beginning an exercise program after a long lay-off period
• Increasing exercise intensity or duration too quickly
• Exercising in worn-out or ill-fitting footwear
• Excessive uphill or downhill running

Biomechanical error: Biomechanical errors are commonly responsible for many chronic injuries and occur when the structures within the body are not functioning as they should.

A common biomechanical error is *muscle imbalance*. This is where one muscle, or group of muscles, is either stronger or more flexible than its opposing muscles. This can occur on the left and right sides of the body, or the front and back of the body.

For example, a right-footed kicker (of any sport that requires kicking) will commonly have overdeveloped quadriceps muscles on the right-hand side, as compared to their left-hand side. This can contribute to a pulling on the right-hand side of the hips and result in chronic pain in the ankle, knee, or lower back.

Other biomechanical errors include:
• Leg length differences
• Tight or stiff muscles
• Foot structure problems, such as flat feet
• Gait or running style problems, such as pronation or supination

Once the underlying cause of the injury has been identified, a conditioning program or training aid can be used to correct the problem. This may involve strength or flexibility exercises in the event of weak or tight muscles. It may involve orthotics or shoe inserts in the case of pronation, supination, or leg length differences. Or it may involve the modification of the athlete's current training program to prevent overload.

Practical

The next section outlines a progressive plan of conditioning exercises, stretches, and drills to fully rehabilitate the injured knee. The progressive plan is arranged so that the individual can choose the right stage to start the process, depending on the extent of the injury. For example, if stages 1, 2, and 3 can be performed without pain, start at stage 4.

Do not progress to the next stage until the current stage can be performed pain free. Of course, some discomfort may be felt, but never push the injured knee to the point where pain or excessive discomfort is experienced.

The progressive plan of exercises below focuses on the knee. However, the last part of the previous section (identifying the underlying causes of injury) must be completed so that other exercises can be incorporated into the rehabilitation program. The knee does not work in isolation from the rest of the body. While the immediate injury may have occurred to the knee, a retraining of the entire body may be necessary to fully rehabilitate and, more importantly, prevent the injury from occurring again.

To personalize and optimize the progressive plan below with exercises specific to your circumstances, you may require the help of a qualified professional, such as a physiotherapist or sports injury rehabilitation specialist. Please consult a professional for specific help with your injury.

Stage 1: Movement-Based Exercises
This stage focuses entirely on simple leg movements. No weight should be placed on the injured leg, and no form of stretching should be used. Simply stand on the uninjured leg, holding onto something for stability if needed, and gently move the injured leg. Exercises could include:
- Lifting the foot up and down
- Swinging the leg back and forth, or side to side
- Making circles with the foot and lower leg
- Flexing and extending the knee

Stage 2: Weight-Bearing and Range of Motion (ROM) Exercises

During this stage a small amount of weight bearing can be applied to the injured knee. Start by simply standing on both legs. When you can comfortably support the weight of your own body, you can progress to walking and stationary cycling. Also incorporate gentle range of motion exercises to lengthen the muscles of the quadriceps and hips.

Stage 3: Isometric Exercises, Gentle Static Stretching

Isometric exercises are exercises where the injured leg does not move, yet force is applied and the muscles of the injured leg are contracted. Start with light or gentle contractions and as the injured leg gets stronger increase the intensity of the contractions. Keep performing these types of exercise until you can do 3 sets of 10 contractions without pain or excessive fatigue.

Another form of exercise to include at this stage is balancing exercise without movement. For example, start with one foot in front of the other, place your arms out to the sides for balance, and hold the position for 15 seconds. Then swap the position of your feet and repeat. If this is easy, try the exercise with your eyes closed.

Also start incorporating gentle static stretching exercises for the muscle groups around the knee. Static stretching is performed by placing the body into a position whereby the muscle (or group of muscles) to be stretched is under tension. Both the opposing muscle group and the muscles to be stretched are relaxed. Then, slowly and cautiously, the body is moved to increase the tension of the stretched muscle group. At this point the position is held or maintained to allow the muscles to lengthen.

Stretching exercises should be included for the lower back, the hips and buttocks, the quadriceps, the hamstrings, the adductors, and the calf muscles.

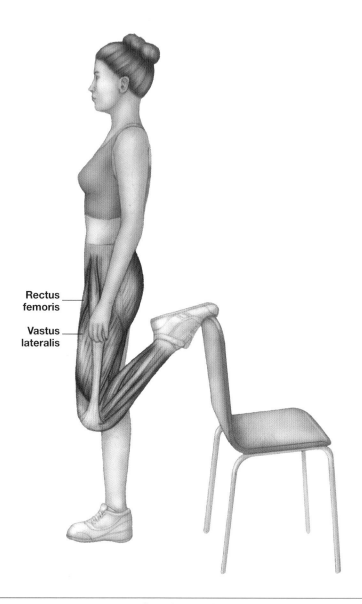

Rectus femoris

Vastus lateralis

Quad stretch

Technique

Stand with your back to a chair and raise your foot up onto the chair. Gently push your hips forward until you can feel tension in the front of your thigh.

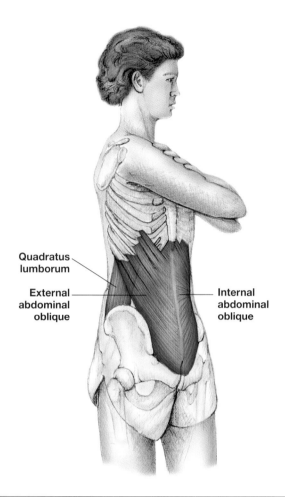

Quadratus lumborum

External abdominal oblique

Internal abdominal oblique

Standing back rotation stretch
Technique

Stand with your feet shoulder-width apart. Place your hands across your chest while keeping your back and shoulders upright. Slowly rotate your shoulders to one side. Repeat.

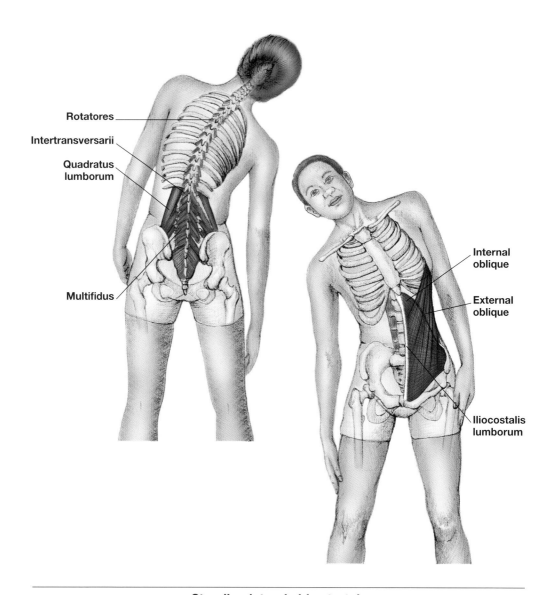

Rotatores

Intertransversarii

Quadratus lumborum

Multifidus

Internal oblique

External oblique

Iliocostalis lumborum

Standing lateral side stretch
Technique

Stand with your feet shoulder-width apart and look forward. Keep your body upright and slowly bend to the left or right. Reach down your leg with your hand and do not bend forward. Do not lean forward or backward.

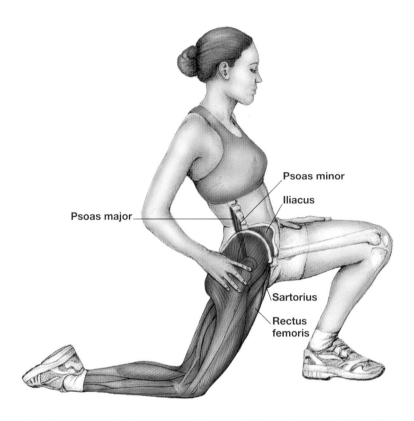

Psoas minor

Iliacus

Psoas major

Sartorius

Rectus femoris

Kneeling quad stretch
Technique
Kneel on one foot and the other knee. If needed, hold onto something to keep your balance. Push your hips forward.

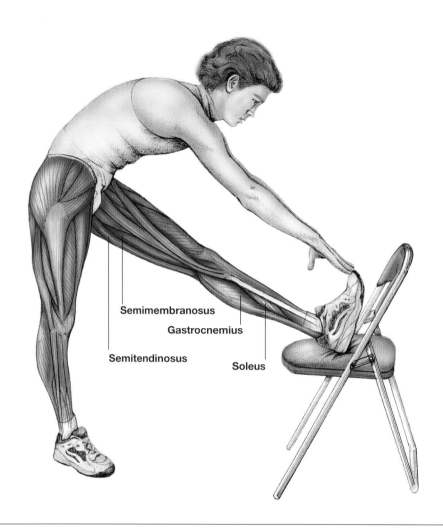

Semimembranosus

Gastrocnemius

Semitendinosus

Soleus

Standing leg-up hamstring stretch
Technique
Stand upright and raise one leg onto an object. Keep that leg straight and your toes pointing straight up.
Lean forward while keeping your back straight.

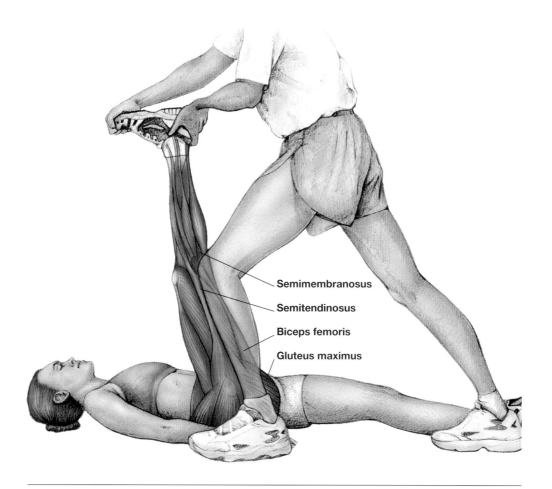

Semimembranosus

Semitendinosus

Biceps femoris

Gluteus maximus

Lying bent knee hamstring stretch

Technique

Lie on your back and bend one leg. Pull the other knee toward
your chest, then slowly and gently straighten your raised leg.

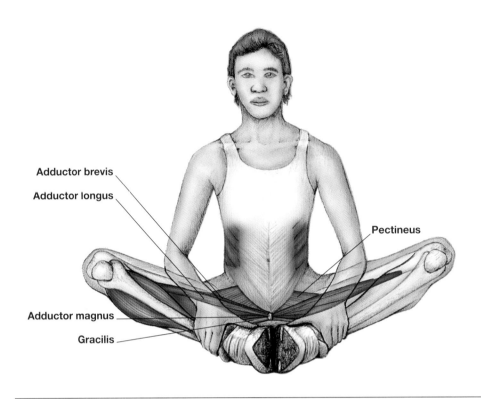

Adductor brevis

Adductor longus

Pectineus

Adductor magnus

Gracilis

Sitting feet together adductor stretch

Technique

Sit with the soles of your feet together and bring your feet toward your groin. Hold onto your ankles and push your knee toward the ground with your elbows. Keep your back straight and upright.

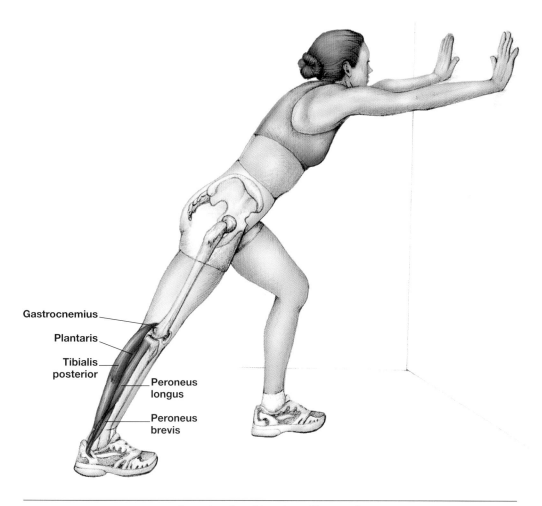

Gastrocnemius

Plantaris

Tibialis posterior

Peroneus longus

Peroneus brevis

Leaning heel back calf stretch

Technique

Stand upright and lean against a wall. Place one foot as far from the wall is as comfortable and make sure that both toes are facing forward and your heel is on the ground. Keep your back leg straight and lean toward the wall.

Stage 4: Movement-Based Strength Training (Assisted and Isolated)

Specific movement-based exercises can now be used to improve the strength of the supporting muscle groups around the knee. It is important to start with assisted, isolated exercises first. An *assisted exercise* is an exercise where a machine, some apparatus, or another person is used to help stabilize the body during the exercise; an *isolated exercise* is an exercise that only involves one muscle group and one joint at a time. Machine-type weights are very helpful here, and common examples of assisted, isolated exercises include the leg extension machine, the hamstring curl machine, and the standing calf raise. Start with a very light weight and work towards 3 sets of 10 repetitions.

Continue to include static stretching exercises for the muscle groups listed in stage 3.

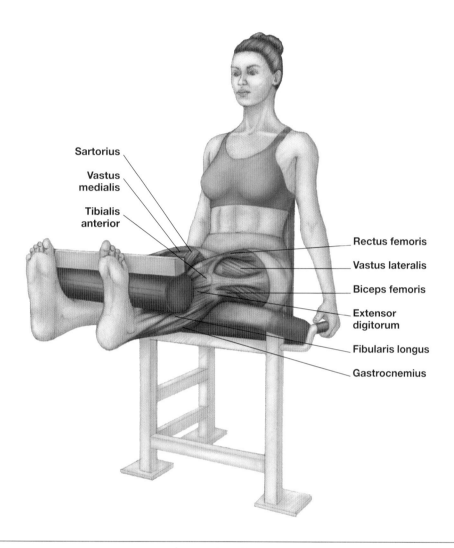

Sartorius

Vastus medialis

Tibialis anterior

Rectus femoris

Vastus lateralis

Biceps femoris

Extensor digitorum

Fibularis longus

Gastrocnemius

Leg extension
Technique

Extend your legs, kicking your feet outwards and up until your knees are completely extended. Allow your lower legs to drop and return to the starting position.

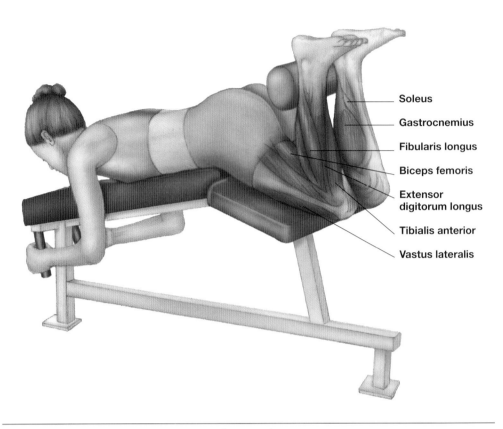

Soleus

Gastrocnemius

Fibularis longus

Biceps femoris

Extensor
digitorum longus

Tibialis anterior

Vastus lateralis

Leg curl
Technique

Contract your hamstrings and pull your heels up and in until the bar comes into contact with your lower glutes or until your knees reach at least 90 degrees of flexion. Lower the weight in a controlled movement.

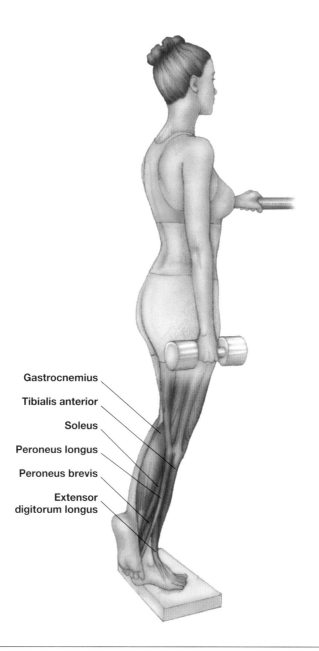

Gastrocnemius

Tibialis anterior

Soleus

Peroneus longus

Peroneus brevis

Extensor
digitorum longus

Calf raise
Technique

With body vertical, place the ball joint to the toe of one or both feet on a step. Either one of both feet should be extended, so that the heel and arch of each foot is beyond the edge of the step. Hips, ankles, shoulders aligned, with spine in neutral position; head up. Use a dumbbell to increase the intensity of the exercise.

Stage 5: Movement-Based Strength Training (Unassisted and Integrated)

Once the exercises in stage 4 can be completed without pain or excessive fatigue, start to incorporate a few unassisted exercises. As opposed to assisted exercises, unassisted exercises are exercises performed without the aid of a machine, some apparatus, or another person for support. This means that only the muscles within your own body are able to provide support while performing an unassisted exercise. Free weights are a good example of unassisted exercises.

This is also the time to incorporate more integrated exercises. *Integrated exercises*, as opposed to isolated exercises, are exercises that involve multiple muscle groups and multiple joints.

Begin with exercises like the leg press and the adductor machine, which are assisted, integrated exercises. Then move on to exercises like squats, lunges (front, back, and side), good mornings, and cable pulls for the adductors and abductors, which are unassisted, integrated exercises. Start off with very light weights and work towards 3 sets of 10 repetitions.

Continue to include static stretching exercises for the muscle groups listed in stage 3. Now, at stage 5 of the rehabilitation, the stretches should be held for 20 to 30 seconds each and a moderate amount of force can be applied to the stretched muscle groups.

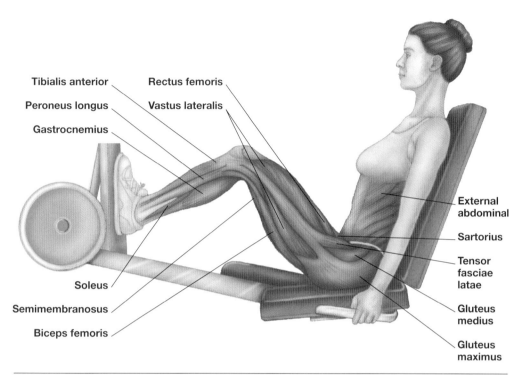

Tibialis anterior
Peroneus longus
Gastrocnemius
Rectus femoris
Vastus lateralis
External abdominal
Sartorius
Tensor fasciae latae
Soleus
Semimembranosus
Biceps femoris
Gluteus medius
Gluteus maximus

Leg press
Technique
Keep legs parallel and push firmly into your foot base, extending both knees and hips simultaneously until your knees are fully extended. Then return to the start position.

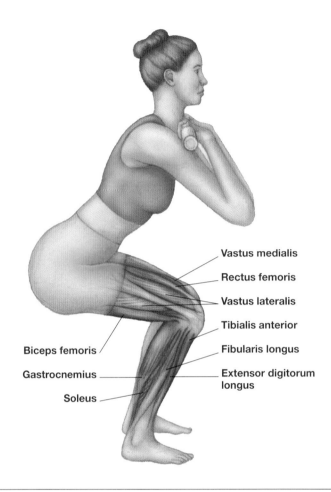

Vastus medialis

Rectus femoris

Vastus lateralis

Tibialis anterior

Biceps femoris

Fibularis longus

Gastrocnemius

Extensor digitorum longus

Soleus

Squats
Technique
Slowly lower the body, moving the hips back as if sitting into a chair. Lower to approximately 90 degrees of knee flexion, i.e. stop before the upper leg becomes parallel with the floor. Return and repeat.

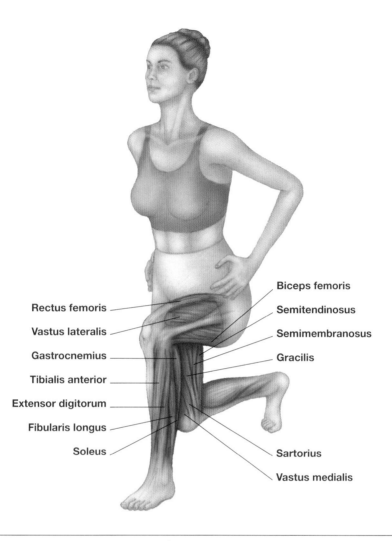

Rectus femoris
Vastus lateralis
Gastrocnemius
Tibialis anterior
Extensor digitorum
Fibularis longus
Soleus

Biceps femoris
Semitendinosus
Semimembranosus
Gracilis

Sartorius
Vastus medialis

Lunges
Technique

Keeping your head up, your spine in neutral, and your hands on your hips, step forward, bending your front knee to a 90-degree angle, and drop your front thigh until it is parallel with the ground. Drop your back knee behind you, so that you are balancing on the toe of your foot to create a 90-degree angle in your knee joint and a straight line from your spine through your bottom knee.

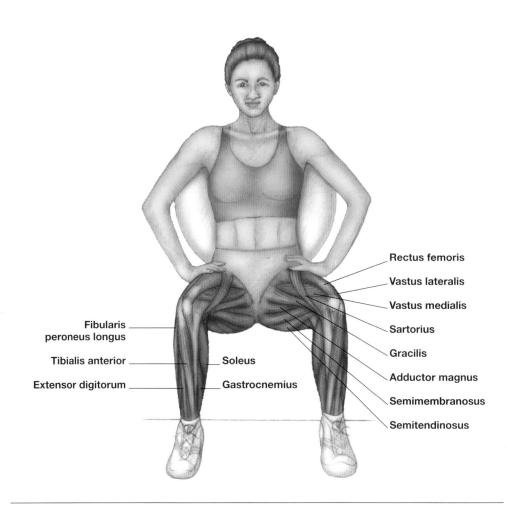

Rectus femoris

Vastus lateralis

Vastus medialis

Fibularis
peroneus longus

Sartorius

Tibialis anterior

Gracilis

Soleus

Adductor magnus

Extensor digitorum

Gastrocnemius

Semimembranosus

Semitendinosus

Wall squat
Technique
Stand with the ball in the curve of your back against the wall. Feet should be shoulder-width apart, stomach scooped, and glutes lightly squeezed. Slowly roll down the wall to a point that is no further than 90 degrees at the knee. Hold the position for ten seconds. Roll back up the ball.

Stage 6: Balance Exercises With Movement, Light PNF Stretching

Once the example exercises in the previous stages can be performed without excessive fatigue and do not result in excessive soreness 24 to 48 hours after they have been completed, continue to perform the exercises with increased weight.

During this stage balancing exercises with movement are added to improve the body's ability to stabilize itself. Walking along a beam and exercises that involve a Swiss ball or wobble board are helpful for this purpose.

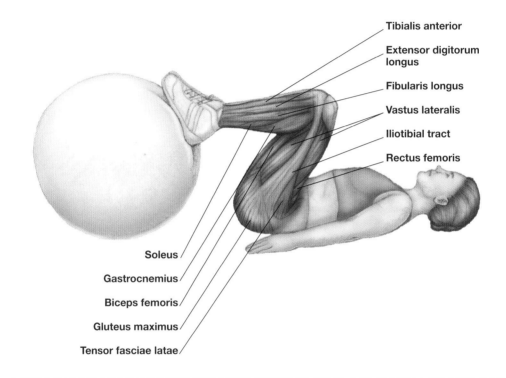

Tibialis anterior

Extensor digitorum longus

Fibularis longus

Vastus lateralis

Iliotibial tract

Rectus femoris

Soleus

Gastrocnemius

Biceps femoris

Gluteus maximus

Tensor fasciae latae

Straight leg bridge
Technique
Start with the ball under your legs and close to your body. By pressing out and down into the ball with the backs of your legs, roll yourself up off the floor until your hips and knees are straight.

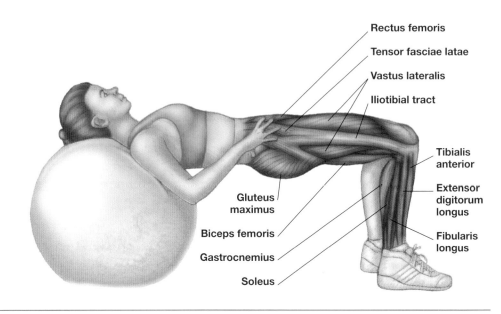

Rectus femoris

Tensor fasciae latae

Vastus lateralis

Iliotibial tract

Tibialis anterior

Extensor digitorum longus

Fibularis longus

Gluteus maximus

Biceps femoris

Gastrocnemius

Soleus

Suspension bridge
Technique
Rest your head and shoulders on the ball, with your stomach scooped in. Do not arch your back; if your back muscles are too rigid, soften your hips and tip your pelvis back towards you.

The introduction of PNF stretching should be incorporated as well. *PNF stretching*, or *proprioceptive neuromuscular facilitation*, is a more advanced form of flexibility training that involves both the stretching and the contraction of the muscle group being targeted. PNF stretching was originally developed as a form of rehabilitation, and for this purpose it is very effective. It is also excellent for targeting specific muscle groups, and, as well as increasing flexibility, it improves muscular strength.

The process of performing a PNF stretch is as follows. The muscle group to be stretched is positioned so that the muscles are stretched and under tension. The individual then contracts the stretched muscle group for 5–6 seconds while a partner, or immovable object, applies sufficient resistance to inhibit movement. *Please note*: the force of contraction should be relevant to the level of conditioning. Start with light contractions and increase the force of the contraction gradually.

The contracted muscle group is then relaxed and a controlled stretch is applied for about 20 to 30 seconds. The muscle group is then allowed 30 seconds to recover and the process is repeated 2–4 times.

Stage 7: Dynamic Strength Training, Moderate PNF Stretching, Light Dynamic Stretching

Dynamic strength exercises are often referred to as *explosive exercises* or *plyometric exercises*. The idea is to continue with all the strength exercises outlined in the previous stages but perform the exercises with more intensity and velocity. As strength improves, and resistance to fatigue and soreness increases, start to incorporate light plyometric exercises. Plyometric exercises are explosive exercises that both lengthen and contract a muscle at the same time. These are called *eccentric muscle contractions* and involve activities such as jumping, hopping, skipping, and bounding.

A Word of Warning!
Dynamic exercises are an intense form of strength training that your body may not be accustomed to. Always start off easy and gradually apply more and more force or intensity.

Continue to use PNF stretching as outlined in the previous stage, and also start to incorporate light dynamic stretching. Dynamic stretching uses a controlled, soft bounce or swinging motion to move a particular body part to the limit of its range of motion. The force of the bounce or swing is gradually increased but should never become radical or uncontrolled.

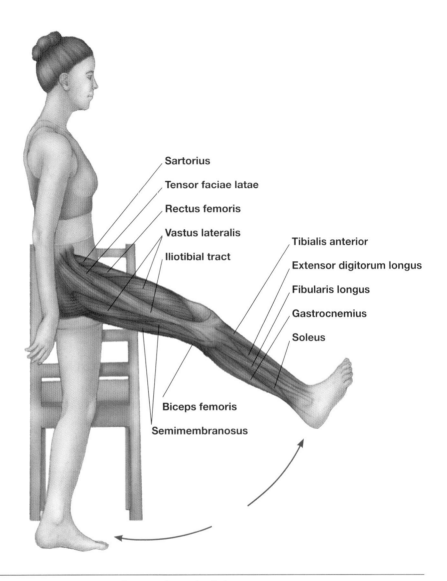

Sartorius

Tensor faciae latae

Rectus femoris

Vastus lateralis

Iliotibial tract

Tibialis anterior

Extensor digitorum longus

Fibularis longus

Gastrocnemius

Soleus

Biceps femoris

Semimembranosus

Leg swing stretch
Technique
Rest your head and shoulders on the ball, with your stomach scooped in. Do not arch your back; if your back muscles are too rigid, soften your hips and tip your pelvis back towards you.

Stage 8: Skill Drills Incorporating Multiple Aspects of Previous Stages, Dynamic Stretching

In this last stage of the rehabilitation process a greater intensity is applied to all the exercises of the previous stages. Continue to work through all the exercises outlined previously, adding more weight, more intensity, more velocity, and more repetitions to them as your strength and fitness improves.

Continue also with more PNF and dynamic stretching, again adding more intensity as your flexibility improves.

Finally, add skill drills and obstacle course-type training to your rehabilitation program. Exercises and drills that relate specifically to your chosen sport are a good place to start.

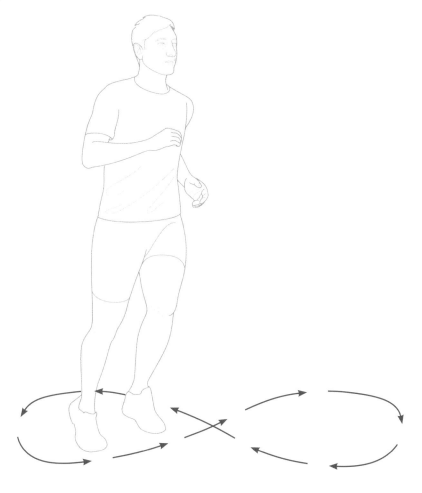

PART III—Knee Injuries and Conditions

Anterior Cruciate Ligament (ACL) Rupture
Biceps Femoris Avulsion Fracture
Bursitis
Chondromalacia Patellae (Runner's Knee)
Fracture: Patellar; Femoral Condyle; Tibial Plateau
Hamstring Rupture
Hamstring Tendinitis
Iliotibial Band (ITB) Syndrome
Knee Joint Dislocation
Knee Plica (Synovial Plica)
Lateral Collateral Ligament (LCL) Rupture
Medial Collateral Ligament (MCL) Rupture
Meniscus Tear
Osgood-Schlatter Syndrome/Disease
Osteoarthritis of the Knee
Osteochondritis Dissecans
Patellar Tendinitis (Jumper's Knee)
Patellar Tendon Rupture
Patellofemoral Pain Syndrome
Popliteus Rupture
Posterior Cruciate Ligament (PCL) Rupture
Quadriceps Contusion (Bruise)
Quadriceps Rupture
Quadriceps Tendinitis
Subluxing Kneecap (Patellar Dislocation)
Tibiofibular Joint Dislocation

Anterior Cruciate Ligament (ACL) Rupture

Classification: Acute

Brief outline of injury

The anterior cruciate ligament (ACL) is one of the four ligaments of the knee and it holds the knee together from the front. An *ACL injury* commonly happens in sports where there are a lot of direction changes and possible impacts. Football, lacrosse, and other fast moving games that require quick changes often result in ACL sprains. The most common mechanism for this injury is when the knee rotates while the foot is planted. Sharp pain at the time of the injury, accompanied by swelling in the knee joint, may be a sign of an ACL tear. This can range from minor tearing of a few fibers to a complete tear. The ACL can also be torn as the result of a hard blow to the knee; usually other ligaments and the meniscus are involved as well.

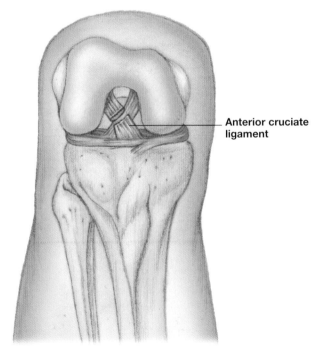

Anterior cruciate ligament

Right leg (anterior view)

Cause of injury
Forceful twisting of the knee when the foot is planted. Occasionally a forceful blow to the knee, especially if the foot is fixed as well.

Signs and symptoms
Pain immediately after injury that may go away later. Swelling in the knee joint. Instability in the knee, especially with the tibia.

Complications if left unattended
If left unattended this injury may not heal properly. The instability in the joint could result in injury of other ligaments. Chronic pain and instability could lead to future limitations.

Immediate treatment
R.I.C.E.R. (immediate referral to a sports medicine professional). Immobilization.

Rehabilitation and prevention
Once stability and strength return and pain subsides, activities such as stationary cycling can be gradually introduced. Range of motion and strengthening exercises are an important part of rehabilitation. Swimming and other exercises that are non-weight bearing may be used until the strength returns to normal. Strengthening the muscles of the quadriceps, hamstrings, and calves will help to protect the ACL. Proper conditioning before beginning high impact activities will also provide protection.

Long-term prognosis and surgery
ACL sprains that involve a complete tear usually require surgery to reattach the ligament. Minor sprains can often be healed completely without surgery. Return to full activity may be a prolonged process and some activities may be limited.

Biceps Femoris Avulsion Fracture

Classification: Acute

Brief outline of injury

An *avulsion fracture* occurs when a tendon or ligament pulls away from the bone at its attachment, pulling a piece of the bone away with it. This usually results from a forceful, twisting muscular contraction or a powerful hyperextension or hyperflexion of the knee. The injury is more prevalent in children than adults: in adults the tendons or ligaments tend to tear before the bone is affected, whereas the softer bones tend to become involved in children's injuries.

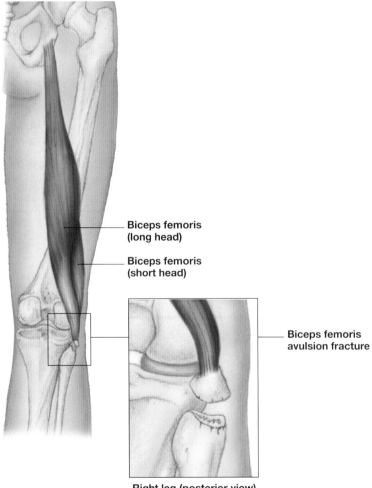

Biceps femoris
(long head)

Biceps femoris
(short head)

Biceps femoris
avulsion fracture

Right leg (posterior view)

Cause of injury
Forceful twisting, extension, or flexion, causing extra stress on the tendon. Direct impact on the knee, causing forceful stretching of the biceps femoris tendon.

Signs and symptoms
Pain at the back of the knee. Swelling and tenderness. Loss of hamstring strength and decreased ability to flex the knee.

Complications if left unattended
When left untreated an avulsion fracture will lead to long-term disability in the hamstrings and knee joint. Incomplete or incorrect healing may result as well, leading to future injuries of the knee and other muscles around the joint.

Immediate treatment
R.I.C.E.R. Immobilization of the knee joint. Anti-inflammatory drugs. Seek immediate medical help.

Rehabilitation and prevention
Rest for the injured knee and then strengthening the muscles and supporting ligaments will help rehabilitate and prevent future fractures. Gradual re-entry into full activity is important to prevent re-injuring the weakened area.

Long-term prognosis and surgery
With proper treatment most simple avulsion fractures will heal completely with no limitations. In rare cases surgery may be needed to repair the avulsed bone, especially in children when the avulsion involves a growth plate.

Bursitis

Classification: Chronic

Brief outline of injury

Bursitis can be a painful condition, especially when located in the weight-bearing knee joint. The job of the bursa is to cushion and lubricate the joint, so if it becomes inflamed, pain will occur in most weight-bearing and flexion or extension activities. With three major bursae surrounding the knee there are many chances to injure one of them. The three major bursae of the knee are the prepatellar bursa, the infrapatellar bursa, and the anserine bursa.

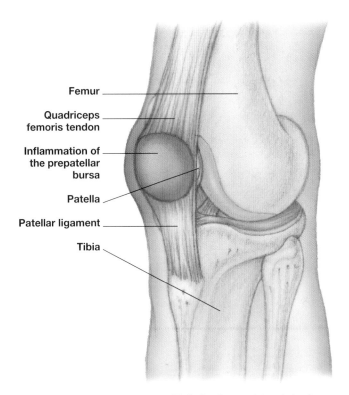

Femur

Quadriceps femoris tendon

Inflammation of the prepatellar bursa

Patella

Patellar ligament

Tibia

Right leg (anterolateral view)

Cause of injury
Repetitive pressure or trauma to the bursa. Repetitive friction between the bursa and tendon or bone.

Signs and symptoms
Pain and tenderness. Mild swelling, due to release of the fluid in the bursal sac. Pain and stiffness when kneeling or when walking down stairs.

Complications if left unattended
The bursa is a fluid-filled sac that is used to lubricate and cushion the joint; if it is allowed to rupture and release the fluid, the natural cushioning will be lost. The build-up of fluid in the joint will cause loss of mobility in the joint as well.

Immediate treatment
R.I.C.E.R. Anti-inflammatory medication.

Rehabilitation and prevention
Strengthening the muscles around the knee helps to support the joint. Increasing flexibility also relieves some of the pressure exerted by the tendons upon the bursa. When a kneeling or crouching position is necessary, frequent rests also help to prevent bursitis. Identifying any underlying problems, such as improper equipment or form, is important during rehabilitation to prevent the condition from recurring.

Long-term prognosis and surgery
Bursitis is seldom a long-term concern if treated properly. Occasional draining of the fluid from the joint is necessary.

Chondromalacia Patellae (Runner's Knee)

Classification: Chronic

Brief outline of injury

The underside of the patella is protected by cartilage. *Chondromalacia patellae* occurs when this cartilage becomes damaged and softens. Softening and degeneration of the cartilage on the underside of the kneecap in athletes is usually a result of overuse, trauma, or abnormal forces on the knee. In older adults it can be a result of degenerative arthritis. Pain under the kneecap and a grating sensation when the knee is extended are possible signs of this condition.

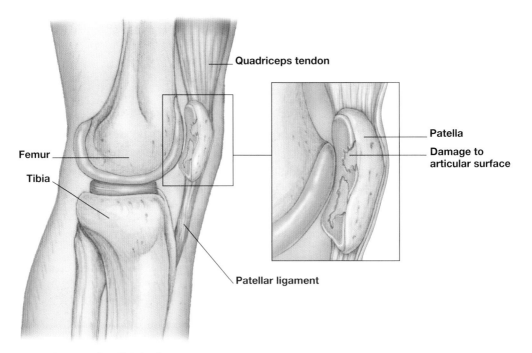

Right leg (medial view)

Cause of injury

Repetitive micro-trauma to the cartilage through overuse conditions. Misalignment of the kneecap. Previous fracture or dislocation of the kneecap.

Signs and symptoms

Pain that worsens after sitting for prolonged periods or when using stairs or rising from a seated position. Tenderness over the kneecap. Grating or grinding sensation when the knee is extended.

Complications if left unattended

Cartilage that degenerates and becomes rough can cause scarring in the bone surface that it rubs against. This in turn causes more inflammation. Cartilage can also be torn when it is rough, leading to loose bodies in the joint.

Immediate treatment

Rest and ice. Anti-inflammatory medications.

Rehabilitation and prevention

Limiting activity until the pain subsides and a gradual reintroduction to the activity is paramount. Strengthening and stretching the quadriceps is important to relieve pressure on the patella. Activities that increase the pain, such as deep knee bending, should be avoided until completely pain free. Avoid abnormal stress on the knee and keep the hamstrings and quadriceps strong and flexible to prevent this condition.

Long-term prognosis and surgery

Chondromalacia patellae commonly responds well to therapy and anti-inflammatory medications. In rare cases surgery may be required to correct a misalignment in the kneecap.

Fracture: Patellar; Femoral Condyle; Tibial Plateau

Classification: Acute

Brief outline of injury

Bones are made of a hard, porous outer shell surrounding softer marrow and blood vessels. When the outer shell is cracked it is called a fracture. The bone may be only partially *fractured* or it may be completely broken. When dealing with the knee, the most commonly involved bones include the patella (kneecap), the femoral condyle, and the tibial plateau. Direct trauma to the knee or twisting force at the knee joint may cause fracturing of these bones. Motor vehicle accidents are the most common cause of these fractures, although contact sports, jumping, and falls can all be causes as well.

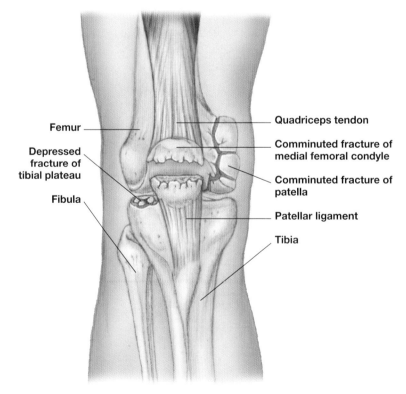

Femur
Depressed fracture of tibial plateau
Fibula

Quadriceps tendon
Comminuted fracture of medial femoral condyle
Comminuted fracture of patella
Patellar ligament
Tibia

Right leg (anterior view)

Cause of injury

Super-high impact across the femur, such as from a car accident or aggressive tackle in football. Direct force (impact) to the bones, such as in a fall or a blow to the lower leg. Rotational or indirect forces on the bones, such as with a tackle in football.

Signs and symptoms

Severe pain, inability to walk or bear weight, and often inability to move the leg. Deformity may be present at the fracture site, or the fracture may be open. Swelling and tenderness. Inability to move the leg or bear weight.

Complications if left unattended

Permanent disability will result if this injury is left untreated. Instability in the lower leg is one long-term complication of an untreated fracture. Blood vessel damage from a fracture can lead to internal bleeding and swelling issues, as well as circulation problems for the foot. Nerve involvement can lead to serious problems such as "drop foot" or loss of sensation in the lower leg and foot.

Immediate treatment

Immobilize the leg, and control any bleeding that might be present with an open fracture. Seek medical attention immediately.

Rehabilitation and prevention

After the fracture has healed it will be necessary to rebuild the strength and flexibility of the muscles in both the upper and the lower leg. Range of motion activities may be needed for the knee, depending on the location of the fracture and the extent of immobilization required. When the fracture has healed a gradual re-entry into activity must be observed to prevent re-injury. Strong calf and tibialis anterior (front of the shin) muscles will help protect the tibia and fibula, while strong quadriceps and hamstrings will help protect the femur.

Long-term prognosis and surgery

If set properly and allowed to heal fully, a knee fracture should not present any future problems. In some cases a rod or pins may be needed to hold the bones in place during healing. Surgery may be required in a few cases where blood vessel, nerve, or ligament damage is severe.

Hamstring Rupture

Classification: Acute

Brief outline of injury

A *hamstring rupture or strain*, or a "pulled hamstring" as it is commonly called, is a stretch or tear of the hamstring muscles and/or tendons. This is a very common injury, especially in activities that involve sprinting or explosive accelerations. A common cause of a hamstring strain is a muscle imbalance between the hamstrings and the quadriceps, with the quadriceps being much stronger. The hamstrings actually consist of three separate muscles that work together to extend the hip and flex the knee. The three muscles of the hamstrings are the *biceps femoris*, *semitendinosus*, and the *semimembranosus*, and any of these can be strained. Commonly, minor tears happen in the belly of the muscle closest to the knee. Complete tears or ruptures usually occur when the muscle pulls away from this attachment as well.

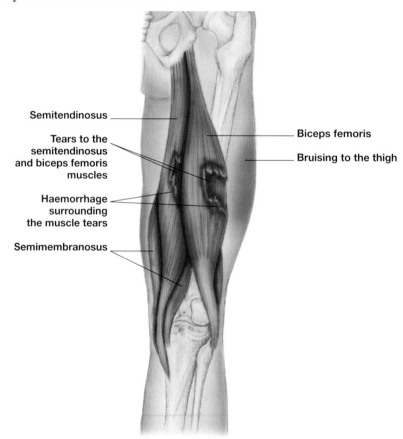

Right leg (posterior view)

Cause of injury
Strength imbalance between the hamstrings and quadriceps. Forceful stretching of the muscle, especially during contraction. Excessive overload on the muscle.

Signs and symptoms
Pain and tenderness in the hamstrings, ranging from very little with a Grade 1 to debilitating with a Grade 3. May affect the ability to walk, causing symptoms ranging from a limp to a complete inability to bear weight. Swelling with Grades 2 and 3.

Complications if left unattended
Pain and tightness in the hamstrings will continue to get worse without treatment. The tightness in the hamstrings could lead to lower back and hip problems. Untreated strains can continue to progress to a complete rupture.

Immediate treatment
Grade 1: Ice, anti-inflammatory medicines.
Grades 2 and 3: R.I.C.E.R., anti-inflammatory medicines, seek medical help if a complete rupture is suspected or if walking unaided is impossible.
Heat, massage and very gentle static stretching can be used after 72 hours to promote blood flow and healing.

Rehabilitation and prevention
Stretching after the initial pain subsides will help speed recovery and prevent future recurrences. Strengthening the hamstrings to balance them with the quadriceps is also important. When restarting activity, a proper warm-up must be stressed and a gradual increase in intensity should be followed.

Long-term prognosis and surgery
Hamstring strains that are fully rehabilitated seldom leave any lingering effects. Complete ruptures may require surgery to repair and long-term rehabilitation.

Hamstring Tendinitis

Classification: Chronic

Brief outline of injury
Hamstring tendinitis, like other versions of tendinitis, involves inflammation of the tendon. This can be a result of repetitive stresses to the hamstring tendons or excessive stress before the muscles are conditioned to cope with it. Pain at the back of the leg above the knee, especially when extending the knee, usually accompanies this injury. Repetitive stress, especially under contraction (such as when accelerating or decelerating), can cause inflammation of the tendons. Minor tears may also occur in the tendon as well when the stress is too much for the tendon to handle.

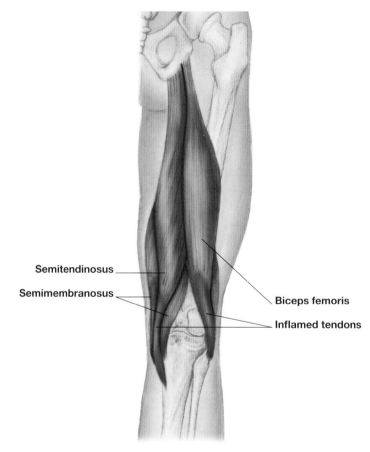

Semitendinosus

Semimembranosus

Biceps femoris

Inflamed tendons

Right leg (posterior view)

Cause of injury
Repetitive stress to the tendons, such as running, jumping, sprinting, etc. Untreated injury to the hamstrings.

Signs and symptoms
Pain at the bottom of the hamstrings, just above the back of the knee joint. Pain is aggravated by jumping, running, and excessive flexion of the knee.

Complications if left unattended
The hamstring muscles may also become inflamed and the tendon will become weak if left untreated. This could lead to a complete rupture of the tendon. A change in gait or landing form can lead to other injuries as well.

Immediate treatment
Rest and ice. Anti-inflammatory medications.

Rehabilitation and prevention
Rehabilitation should include stretching and strengthening exercises for the hamstrings. Activities such as swimming can be helpful to reduce the stress on the tendon during rehabilitation. Return to a normal activity schedule should be delayed until pain subsides completely and strength is restored. Keeping the hamstrings and lower back flexible and strong will help prevent this condition.

Long-term prognosis and surgery
A full recovery with no long-term disability or lingering effects can be expected in most cases of tendinitis. Surgery is only necessary in extremely rare cases of the condition.

Iliotibial Band (ITB) Syndrome

Classification: Chronic

Brief outline of injury

Iliotibial band syndrome is caused by excessive friction between the iliotibial band (or tract) and the lateral epicondyle, at the end of the femur where it forms the knee. This friction can also occur at the hip as well. The friction causes inflammation and pain in the iliotibial band. Since this band of tissue crosses over the bony prominences whenever the knees and hips flex or extend, the condition can be a very painful. The iliotibial band is actually the connective tissue for the tensor fasciae latae muscle: the band attaches to the hip at the top, crosses the knee, and attaches to the tibia at the bottom. If the iliotibial band becomes inflamed due to excessive irritation from the friction when crossing over the bone, it will cause pain and tightness.

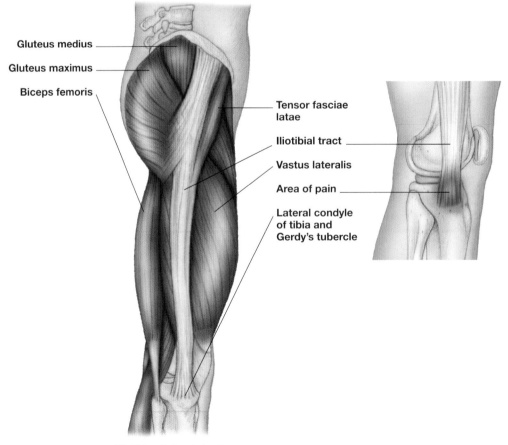

Gluteus medius

Gluteus maximus

Biceps femoris

Tensor fasciae latae

Iliotibial tract

Vastus lateralis

Area of pain

Lateral condyle of tibia and Gerdy's tubercle

Right leg (lateral view)

Cause of injury

Repetitive hip and knee flexion and extension while the tensor fasciae latae is contracted, such as with running or cycling. A tight tensor fasciae latae muscle and iliotibial band. Muscle imbalances.

Signs and symptoms

Pain on the lateral side of the knee over the lateral epicondyle of the femur. Pain with flexion and extension of the knee.

Complications if left unattended

The iliotibial band and accompanying tensor fasciae latae become tight due to the pain and inflammation. If left unattended this can lead to chronic pain and injuries to the knee and/or hip.

Immediate treatment

R.I.C.E.R. Anti-inflammatory medications. Then heat and massage to promote blood flow and healing.

Rehabilitation and prevention

Increasing flexibility as pain allows will help speed recovery. After pain has subsided, increasing strength and flexibility of all the muscles of the thighs and hips to develop balance will help prevent future issues. Identifying and fixing any errors in running form will also help to prevent recurrence of the injury.

Long-term prognosis and surgery

Iliotibial band syndrome can be treated successfully with no lingering effects. Inflammation and pain may return when the activity is resumed, and corrections of form must be made to prevent future problems.

Knee Joint Dislocation

Classification: Acute

Brief outline of injury

A *knee joint dislocation* is a serious injury and quite often involves damage to a number of the structures of the knee, including ligaments, tendons, and menisci. There is also a chance that damage will occur to the vascular structures around the knee, which may require emergency surgery. Dislocation occurs when the top of the tibia (shin bone) is completely dislodged from the end of the femur (thigh bone). A dislocation of the knee joint is most commonly caused by a high impact injury, such as an automobile accident or a severe fall.

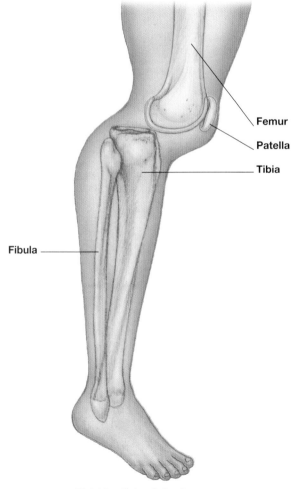

Femur

Patella

Tibia

Fibula

Right leg (lateral view)

Cause of injury
High impact to the knee or leg. Forceful twisting of the knee.

Signs and symptoms
Severe pain. Visible deformity at the joint.

Complications if left unattended
Dislocation of the knee joint causes tearing of the ligaments that hold the joint together. Dislocation results in gross instability and the knee joint becoming considerably more prone to successive dislocations and other injuries.

Immediate treatment
Ice and immobilization. Seek medical attention immediately.

Rehabilitation and prevention
During rehabilitation, activities that do not aggravate the injury should be sought, such as swimming and cycling instead of weight-bearing activities like running and walking. Strengthening the muscles around the knee will help to provide support. A knee brace may also be used to provide extra support when initially returning to activity.

Long-term prognosis and surgery
Even if the knee joint relocates without treatment, which is rare, there will still be significant damage to the soft tissues around the joint. In most cases the knee joint will need to be relocated by a physician or medical professional, and as damage to the soft tissues is always present with a knee dislocation, further surgery may be required to fix the soft tissue damage. Extensive rehabilitation is usually required after surgery.

Knee Plica (Synovial Plica)

Classification: Chronic

Brief outline of injury

The *plica* is a thin fibrous membrane that is left over from the fetal knee development. This plica once divided the knee into three separate compartments during fetal development but then became a part of the knee structure as the compartments became one protective cavity. When friction or a pinching between the femur and patella occurs, the plica may become inflamed, causing it to thicken, which in turn causes more friction, creating a vicious cycle. This is common when the knee is flexed and placed under stress.

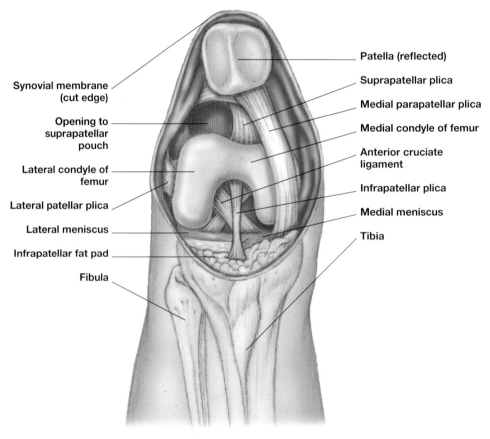

Right leg (anterior view)

Cause of injury

Trauma to the flexed knee. Repetitive stress, especially with medial weight bearing such as in cycling.

Signs and symptoms

Pain. Tenderness over the plica.

Complications if left unattended

The plica will continue to become inflamed and limit flexion activity in the knee if the condition is left unattended. The pain may also cause a change in gait or running form that could lead to other overuse injuries.

Immediate treatment

Reduction of activity. R.I.C.E.R. Anti-inflammatory medication.

Rehabilitation and prevention

Strengthening the quadriceps and hamstrings will take pressure off the plica. Increasing flexibility in these muscles will also relieve pressure that may be irritating the condition. Use of proper equipment, especially running shoes, can eliminate the irritation and force the knee back into proper alignment during activity.

Long-term prognosis and surgery

Once pain subsides a return to normal activity can be expected. Very rarely is arthroscopic surgery required to remove the plica. No adverse effects have been found from the removal of the plica, and a complete return to activity can be expected.

Lateral Collateral Ligament (LCL) Rupture

Classification: Acute

Brief outline of injury

A ligament is tough, fibrous connective tissue that provides support and strength to a joint. A *lateral collateral ligament (LCL) rupture* (as opposed to an MCL rupture) involves tearing or stretching of this ligament of the knee. This ligament is designed to hold the knee joint together on the lateral (outside) surface. Force applied to the inside of the knee causes the outside of the knee to open, stretching the LCL. The extent of the stretch determines whether the ligament simply stretches, tears partially, or tears completely. An LCL rupture is much less common than an MCL rupture.

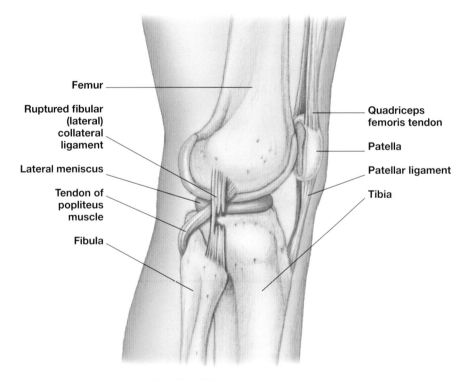

Femur

Ruptured fibular (lateral) collateral ligament

Lateral meniscus

Tendon of popliteus muscle

Fibula

Quadriceps femoris tendon

Patella

Patellar ligament

Tibia

Right leg (lateral view)

Cause of injury
Force applied to the medial side (inside) of the knee joint.

Signs and symptoms
Pain over the lateral portion of the knee. Swelling and tenderness. Instability in the knee and pain with weight bearing.

Complications if left unattended
The ligament, in rare cases, may repair itself if left unattended, but the injury could develop into a more severe rupture. The pain in the knee and instability of the joint may not go away. Continued activity on the injured knee could lead to injuries of the other ligaments, due to the instability.

Immediate treatment
R.I.C.E.R. Immobilization. Anti-inflammatory medication.

Rehabilitation and prevention
Depending on the severity of the rupture, simple rest and gradual introduction back to activity may be enough. For more severe ruptures, braces may be needed during the strengthening phase of rehabilitation and the early portion of the return to activity. The most severe ruptures may require extended immobilization and rest from the activity. As range of motion and strength begins to return, stationary bikes and other equipment may be used to ease back into activity. Ensuring adequate strength in the thigh muscles, and conditioning before starting any activity where the risk of hits to the knee is high, will help prevent these types of injury.

Long-term prognosis and surgery
The ligament will usually heal with no limitations, although in some cases there is residual "looseness" in the lateral part of the knee. Very rarely is surgery required to repair the ligaments. Meniscus tearing that requires surgical repair may also result from an LCL rupture.

Medial Collateral Ligament (MCL) Rupture

Classification: Acute

Brief outline of injury

A *medial collateral ligament (MCL) sprain* involves tearing or stretching of this ligament of the knee. The MCL is one of the most common structures of the knee to be injured. This ligament is designed to hold the knee joint together on the medial (inside) surface. Force applied to the outside of the knee (as in a football tackle) causes the inside of the knee to open, stretching the MCL. The extent of the stretch determines whether the ligament simply stretches, tears partially, or tears completely.

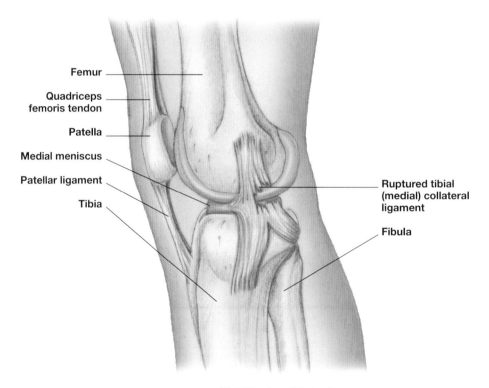

Femur
Quadriceps femoris tendon
Patella
Medial meniscus
Patellar ligament
Tibia
Ruptured tibial (medial) collateral ligament
Fibula

Right leg (medial view)

Cause of injury
Force applied to the lateral side (outside) of the knee joint.

Signs and symptoms
Pain over the medial portion of the knee. Swelling and tenderness. Instability in the knee and pain with weight bearing.

Complications if left unattended
The ligament, in rare cases, may repair itself if left unattended, but the injury could lead to a more severe sprain. The pain in the knee and instability of the joint may not go away. Continued activity on the injured knee could lead to injuries of the other ligaments, due to the instability.

Immediate treatment
R.I.C.E.R. Immobilization. Anti-inflammatory medication.

Rehabilitation and prevention
Depending on the severity of the rupture, simple rest and gradual introduction back to activity may be enough. For more severe ruptures, braces may be needed during the strengthening phase of rehabilitation and the early portion of the return to activity. The most severe rupture may require extended immobilization and rest from the activity. As range of motion and strength begins to return, stationary bikes and other equipment may be used to ease back into activity. Ensuring adequate strength in the thigh muscles, and conditioning before starting any activity where the risk of hits to the knee is high, will help prevent these types of injury.

Long-term prognosis and surgery
The ligament will usually heal with no limitations, although in some cases there is residual "looseness" in the medial part of the knee. Very rarely is surgery required to repair the ligaments. Meniscus tearing that requires surgical repair may also result from an MCL rupture.

Meniscus Tear

Classification: Acute

Brief outline of injury

The meniscus is the cartilage that cushions the knee joint and helps to distribute the weight evenly through the joint. It is attached to the top of the tibia and provides protection for the ends of the femur and tibia where they come together to form the knee. A *meniscus tear* can occur with forceful twisting of the knee, or it may accompany other injuries such as ligament sprains. The "unhappy triad" refers to an injury when a blow to the lateral side of the knee causes tearing of the MCL, the ACL, and the meniscus. This is often seen in sports that require a planting of the foot to quickly change direction.

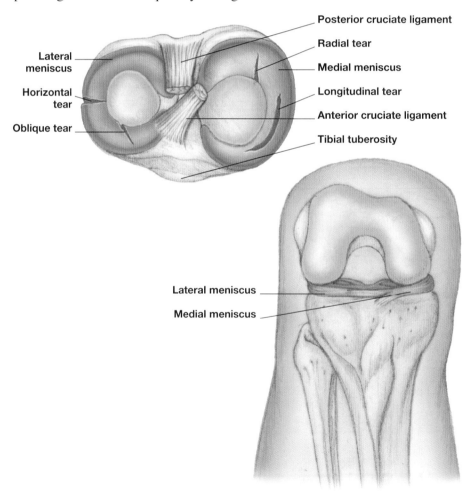

Right leg (anterior view)

Cause of injury
Forceful twisting of the knee joint, most commonly seen when the knee is also bent. May accompany ligament strains as well.

Signs and symptoms
Pain in the knee joint. Some swelling may be noted. Catching, or locking, in the joint.

Complications if left unattended
The loose bodies and jagged edges of a meniscal tear can cause premature wear on the cartilage at the ends of the bones and under the patella. This can lead to arthritic conditions and a fluid build-up in the knee joint.

Immediate treatment
R.I.C.E.R. Anti-inflammatory medications.

Rehabilitation and prevention
After repair of a meniscal tear, it is important to strengthen the muscles surrounding the knee to prevent the injury from happening again. Strong quadriceps and hamstrings help support the knee and prevent the twisting that might cause a tear. The muscles should be stretched regularly as well, since tight muscles can also cause problems in the knee. After a repair, weight bearing should be encouraged where tolerable, but as with any restart of activity it should be done gradually.

Long-term prognosis and surgery
A tear of the meniscus usually requires arthroscopic surgery to repair. The surgery requires removal of the torn edges of the meniscus but leaves the main body of the meniscus intact. Therefore, most meniscus tears heal fully with no long-term limitations.

Osgood-Schlatter Syndrome/Disease

Classification: Chronic

Brief outline of injury

Osgood-Schlatter syndrome/disease is a condition that affects young teens. It is more prevalent in males than females and has a slightly higher prevalence in the left knee than the right. The patella tendon pulls on the tibial tuberosity just below the knee, and when the quadriceps are tight or repetitive flexion and extension is present, this stress may cause small avulsion fractures, resulting in inflammation and pain. Active children or those with previous knee injuries are more susceptible to this condition. During running, jumping, and kicking activities, the quadriceps must contract and relax continuously, which also stresses the attachment at the tibia.

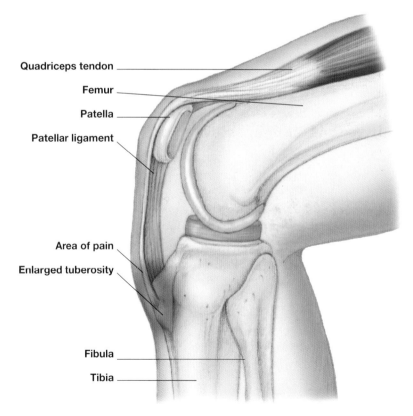

Quadriceps tendon
Femur
Patella
Patellar ligament
Area of pain
Enlarged tuberosity
Fibula
Tibia

Right leg (lateral view)

Cause of injury
Tight quadriceps due to growth spurt. Prior knee injury. Repetitive contractions of the quadriceps muscles.

Signs and symptoms
Pain, worse at full extension and during squatting, subsides with rest. Swelling over the tibial tuberosity, just under the knee. Redness and inflammation of the skin just below the knee.

Complications if left unattended
If left unattended the condition will continue to cause pain and inflammation and could lead to muscle loss in the quadriceps. In rare cases, untreated Osgood-Schlatter syndrome could lead to a complete avulsion fracture of the tibia.

Immediate treatment
R.I.C.E.R. Anti-inflammatory medications.

Rehabilitation and prevention
Most cases of Osgood-Schlatter syndrome respond well to rest that is followed by a regimen of stretching and strengthening of the quadriceps muscles. Limiting activities that cause pain and tend to aggravate the issue is important during recovery. Gradual increases in intensity and proper warm-up techniques will help prevent this condition.

Long-term prognosis and surgery
This condition tends to correct itself as the bone becomes stronger and mature. The pain and inflammation go away and there are seldom any long-term effects. Rare cases may require corticosteroid injections to aid recovery.

Osteoarthritis of the Knee

Classification: Chronic

Brief outline of injury

Osteoarthritis, or *degenerative joint disease*, is a progressive degenerative disease that wears away at the joint cartilage, which is a stiff connective tissue that allows for smooth movement as the knee joint flexes and extends, and which also acts as a shock absorber. As osteoarthritis progresses, the protective cartilage becomes thin and, in extreme cases, the ends of the bones can be exposed. Osteoarthritis of the knee is more common in patients who are over 50 and overweight.

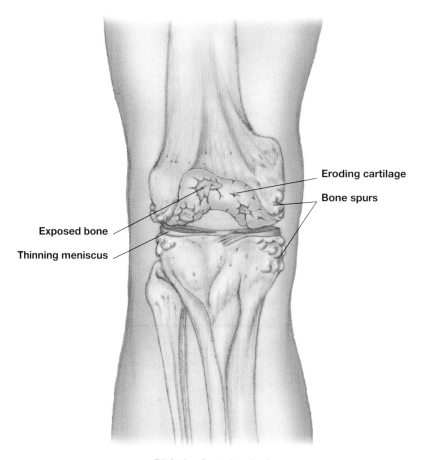

Eroding cartilage

Bone spurs

Exposed bone

Thinning meniscus

Right leg (anterior view)

Cause of injury

Long-term repetitive overuse. Excessive weight or overloading of the knee joint. Previous injury to the knee, such as a fracture or a meniscus injury.

Signs and symptoms

Pain, swelling, and tenderness, especially during activity. Stiffness and limited range of motion. Crunching, grinding, and locking of the knee joint.

Complications if left unattended

If left unattended the cartilage will degenerate to the point where the ends of the bones will be grinding on each other, at which point surgery will be the only option for relief.

Immediate treatment

Rest and ice. Anti-inflammatory medications.

Rehabilitation and prevention

Osteoarthritis is an extremely difficult condition to reverse, so prevention is a high priority. All efforts should be made to reduce any excess body weight and modify any activities that put repeated stress on the knee joint. Improving the condition of the muscles around the knee with strengthening and stretching exercises will provide added support to the knee joint. Another alternative is to take glucosamine supplements, which may help to prevent further degeneration of the cartilage, and may even help to rebuild it. Please note: research into glucosamine supplementation is limited.

Long-term prognosis and surgery

If prevention strategies are not initiated at an early stage, osteoarthritis of the knee may progress to the point where surgery is the only option. Depending on the severity of the condition, and the overall health of the patient, a number of surgical options are available. These range from knee arthroscopy, where the surgeon uses fiber-optic technology to look inside the joint and clean it of debris, to a total knee replacement.

Osteochondritis Dissecans

Classification: Acute or chronic

Brief outline of injury

Osteochondritis dissecans (loose bodies in the joint) results from a loss of blood supply to the bone end and the cartilage covering it. This causes the cartilage to become brittle and a piece, or several pieces, may break off. If this happens and a piece gets into the joint, it can cause pain and inflammation. Although this condition can also happen in the ankle or elbow, it most commonly affects the knee.

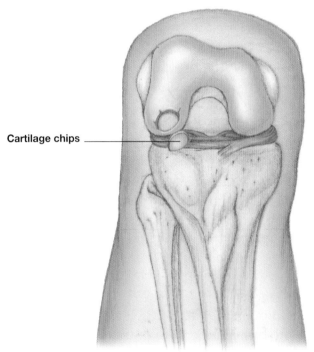

Right leg (anterior view)

Cause of injury
Loss of blood supply to the end of the bone and attached cartilage. Impact to the joint causing a tearing or breaking of the cartilage at the bone end. Repetitive friction leading to the cartilage becoming brittle and breaking away.

Signs and symptoms
Pain, especially during activity. Stiffness with rest. Clicking, locking, or weakness in the joint

Complications if left unattended
If left unattended the loose bodies will continue to cause damage to the inner surface of the joint and could eventually lead to degenerative osteoarthritis. The loose bodies could also lead to tearing or "grooving" of other cartilage in the joint.

Immediate treatment
Rest and referral to a sports medicine professional. Immobilization. Anti-inflammatory medications.

Rehabilitation and prevention
Strengthening the muscles surrounding the affected joint will help support it better during activity. Limiting the amount of time spent doing repetitive movements with the joint may also be required. Treatment of minor injuries to the joint may also help stop the chance of the blood supply being cut off. Limit activities that cause pain and gradually work back into a full schedule.

Long-term prognosis and surgery
If the broken cartilage does not release from the bone it may repair itself, but if it becomes lodged in the joint and the body does not dissolve it, surgery may be required. In younger athletes a complete recovery and return to activity may be expected. In older athletes the development of degenerative osteoarthritis is usually a by-product of this condition.

Patellar Tendinitis (Jumper's Knee)

Classification: Chronic

Brief outline of injury

Activities that require repetitive jumping like basketball or volleyball can lead to *patellar tendinitis*, also referred to as *jumper's knee*, which is tendinitis in the patellar tendon. The tendon is forced to stretch as the quadriceps contract to slow down the flexion of the knee. This repetitive stress can lead to minor trauma in the tendon, which will lead to inflammation. Repetitive flexing and extending of the knee also places stress on this tendon if the tendon does not travel in the required path. The pain is generally felt just below the kneecap.

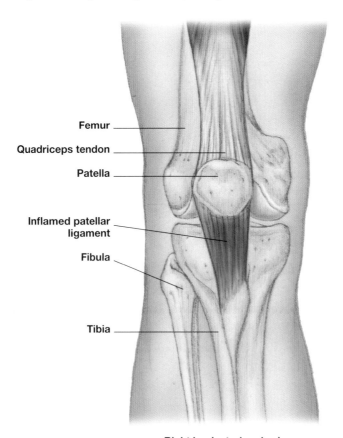

Femur
Quadriceps tendon
Patella
Inflamed patellar ligament
Fibula
Tibia

Right leg (anterior view)

Cause of injury
Repetitive jumping and landing activities. Running and kicking activities can also cause this condition. Untreated minor injury of the patellar tendon.

Signs and symptoms
Pain over the patellar tendon, especially during activity or kneeling. Swelling and tenderness around the tendon.

Complications if left unattended
As with most tendinitis, inflammation that is left untreated will cause additional irritation, which causes more inflammation, setting up a vicious cycle. This can eventually lead to a rupture of the tendon. Damage to surrounding tissue may also happen.

Immediate treatment
R.I.C.E.R. Anti-inflammatory medications.

Rehabilitation and prevention
Stretching the quadriceps, hamstrings, and calves will help relieve pressure on the patellar tendon. During rehabilitation it is important to identify the conditions that caused the injury in the first place. Thorough warm-ups and proper conditioning can help prevent the onset of this condition. A support strap placed below the knee may be needed at first, to support the tendon during the initial return to activity. Prevention of this condition requires strong quadriceps and a good strength balance between the muscles that surround the knee.

Long-term prognosis and surgery
Complete recovery without lingering effects can be expected with good treatment of this condition. Occasionally, the condition may return due to a weakened tendon, especially in older athletes.

Patellar Tendon Rupture

Classification: Acute

Brief Outline of Injury

A *patellar tendon rupture* is a stretch or tear of the tendon that connects the distal end of the patella (bottom of the knee cap) to the front of the tibia (shin bone). The patellar tendon continues around and past the knee cap and connects to the quadriceps muscle. When the quadriceps muscle contracts it pulls on the patellar tendon, which extends (straightens) the knee joint. A patellar tendon rupture can result from a forceful contraction of the quadriceps. As with other strains or ruptures it is graded 1 through 3, with 3 being the most severe.

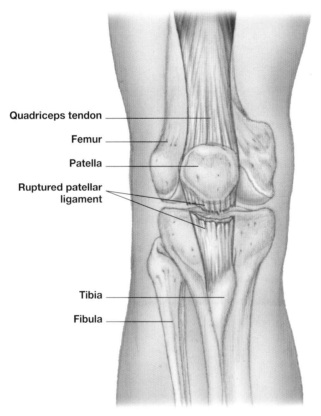

Quadriceps tendon

Femur

Patella

Ruptured patellar ligament

Tibia

Fibula

Right leg (anterior view)

Cause of injury
Forceful contraction of the quadriceps, especially eccentric contractions in which the muscle both contracts and lengthens at the same time, such as when landing from a jump.

Signs and symptoms
Grade 1: Mild pain just below the knee cap, little or no swelling, with very little loss of function of the knee joint. Grade 2: More marked pain and tenderness, moderate swelling, and noticeable strength and stability loss at the knee joint. Grade 3 (full tear): Extreme pain, misalignment or excessive movement of the knee cap, inability to stand or bear weight.

Complications if left unattended
A Grade 1 or Grade 2 rupture left unattended can continue to tear and become worse. A Grade 3 rupture left untreated will result in a loss of function and stability in the knee.

Immediate treatment
R.I.C.E.R. Anti-inflammatory medications. Immobilization in severe cases.

Rehabilitation and prevention
The patellar tendon receives very little blood supply so recovery can be a long process. After the required rest period, activities should be approached cautiously. For most Grade 1 and Grade 2 ruptures, stretching and strengthening the quadriceps will be necessary. Balancing exercises will also help to strengthen the structures of the knee joint. Proper warm-up techniques must be observed to prevent further ruptures, and gradually increasing intensity will help as well. Avoid activities that cause pain.

Long-term prognosis and surgery
Most Grade 1 and Grade 2 ruptures respond well to the above treatment and will seldom result in any long-term pain or disability. However, a Grade 3 rupture will require surgery to reattach the torn tendon.

Patellofemoral Pain Syndrome

Classification: Chronic

Brief outline of injury

Pain in the kneecap, especially after sitting for a long time or running downhill, may be due to a fairly common condition called *patellofemoral pain syndrome*. The pain may result from incorrect movement of the patella over the femur or from tight tendons. The cartilage under the kneecap may become inflamed as well, leading to another condition called *chondromalacia patellae*.

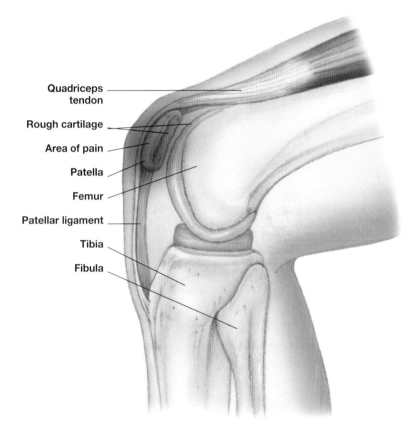

Quadriceps tendon
Rough cartilage
Area of pain
Patella
Femur
Patellar ligament
Tibia
Fibula

Right leg (lateral view)

Cause of injury
Incorrect running form or improper shoes. Weak or tight quadriceps. Chronic patella dislocations.

Signs and symptoms
Pain on and under the kneecap, which worsens after sitting for extended periods or walking down stairs. Clicking or grinding may be felt when flexing the knee.

Complications if left unattended
The inflammation from this condition if left unattended can worsen and cause more permanent damage to the surrounding structures. If the tendon becomes inflamed it could eventually lead to rupture. The cartilage under the patella may also become inflamed.

Immediate treatment
Rest – this can be simply reducing the intensity and duration. Ice and anti-inflammatory medications.

Rehabilitation and prevention
Rehabilitation starts with restoring the strength and flexibility of the quadriceps. When returning to activity after the pain has subsided, gradual increases in intensity, limiting repetitive stresses on the knee, and proper warm-up techniques will ensure that the pain does not return. Strong, flexible quadriceps and hamstrings and avoiding overuse issues will help prevent patellofemoral pain syndrome. A good warm-up before training will also help.

Long-term prognosis and surgery
With complete treatment there are seldom any long-lasting effects. If the condition does not respond to treatment, surgical intervention may be necessary.

Popliteus Rupture

Classification: Acute

Brief outline of injury

A *popliteus rupture*, or strain, is a stretch or tear of the popliteus muscle and/ or tendon. The popliteus is a small muscle located at the back of the knee and helps to initiate flexion of the knee. This muscle is commonly injured when an athlete lands with a fully extended (straight) leg and the knee is forced into hyperextension.

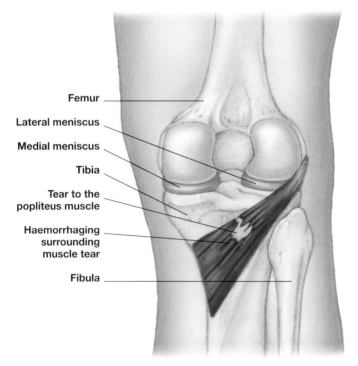

Right leg (posterior view)

Cause of injury
Forceful stretching of the muscle, especially during contraction. Excessive overload on the muscle.

Signs and symptoms
Pain and tenderness in the area directly behind the knee. Discomfort when trying to straighten the knee. May affect the ability to walk, causing symptoms ranging from a limp to a complete inability to bear weight.

Complications if left unattended
Pain and tightness in the popliteus will continue to get worse without treatment. Untreated minor strains can progress to a full rupture.

Immediate treatment
Grade 1: Rest, ice, anti-inflammatory medicines.
Grades 2 and 3: R.I.C.E.R., anti-inflammatory medicines, seek medical help if a complete rupture is suspected or if there is an inability to walk without aid.

Rehabilitation and prevention
Heat, massage, and gentle static stretching after the initial pain subsides will help speed recovery and prevent future recurrences. Strengthening all the muscles at the back of the leg (hamstrings and calf muscles) is also important. When restarting activity, a proper warm-up must be stressed and a gradual increase in intensity should be followed.

Long-term prognosis and surgery
Popliteus ruptures that are fully rehabilitated seldom leave any lingering effects. Complete ruptures and avulsion fractures of the popliteus tendon may require surgery to repair and long-term rehabilitation.

Posterior Cruciate Ligament (PCL) Rupture

Classification: Acute

Brief outline of injury

The posterior cruciate ligament (PCL) is one of the four ligaments of the knee and it holds the knee together from the rear. A *PCL injury* commonly occurs in sports such as soccer, hockey, and football, where there is a high risk of impact to the tibia or lower leg, especially when the knee is bent. Injury to the PCL can range from minor tearing of a few fibers to a complete rupture, and it is often damaged in conjunction with other knee structures. The PCL is less commonly injured compared to the ACL.

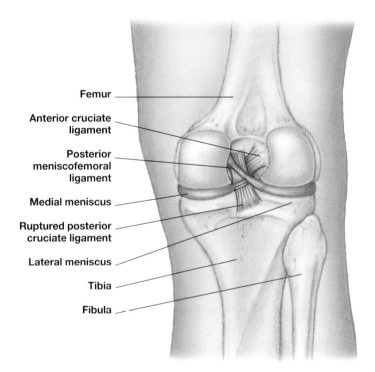

Femur

Anterior cruciate ligament

Posterior meniscofemoral ligament

Medial meniscus

Ruptured posterior cruciate ligament

Lateral meniscus

Tibia

Fibula

Right leg (posterior view)

Cause of injury
Forceful impact to the tibia when the foot is planted and the knee flexed.

Signs and symptoms
Pain in the knee joint at the time of impact. Swelling in the knee joint. Instability in the knee or a feeling of the knee giving out.

Complications if left unattended
If left unattended this injury may not heal properly. The instability in the joint could lead to injury to other ligaments. Chronic pain and instability could lead to future limitations.

Immediate treatment
R.I.C.E.R. (immediate referral to a sports medicine professional). Immobilization.

Rehabilitation and prevention
Once stability and strength return and pain subsides, activities such as stationary cycling can be gradually introduced. Range of motion and strengthening exercises are an important part of rehabilitation. Swimming and other exercises that are non-weight bearing may be used until the strength returns to normal. Strengthening the muscles of the quadriceps, hamstrings, and calves will help to protect the PCL. Proper conditioning before beginning high impact activities will also provide protection.

Long-term prognosis and surgery
If the damage is minor (Grade 1) and no other structures within the knee have been injured, a full recovery can be expected. Minor sprains can usually be healed completely without surgery. PCL ruptures that involve a complete tear often require surgery to reattach the ligament. Return to full activity may be a prolonged process and some activities may be limited.

Quadriceps Contusion (Bruise)

Classification: Acute

Brief outline of injury
A *thigh contusion* is actually a deep bruise of the muscles of the quadriceps near the femur. An impact to any of these muscles squeezes the muscle between the impacting force and the femur. The bruising causes pain and limited flexibility in the muscle. High impact sports such as football or hockey are commonly associated with thigh bruising, but any activity that could result in falling on the thigh or getting hit in that region can cause a contusion.

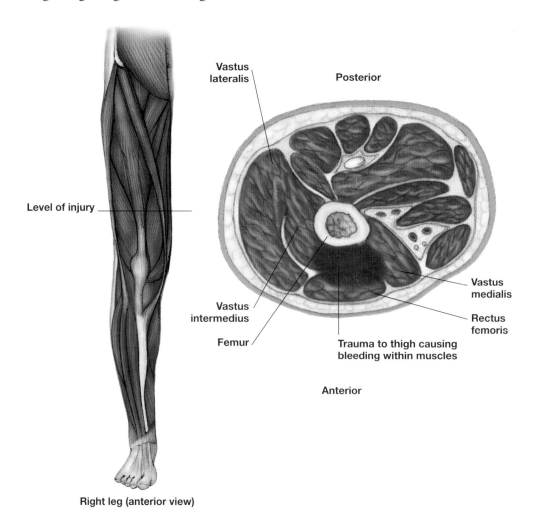

Right leg (anterior view)

Cause of injury
Impact to the muscle from a blunt surface such as the ground, a helmet, a foot, etc.

Signs and symptoms
Pain and tenderness over the injured area. Swelling and bruising may be present. Pain with weight bearing and stretching of the muscle

Complications if left unattended
Myositis ossificans, which is the formation of bone in the muscle tissue, can develop from unattended thigh contusions. Muscle ruptures can also occur when a contusion is left untreated and activity is continued.

Immediate treatment
Rest and ice. Anti-inflammatory medications. Then heat, massage and very gentle static stretching to promote blood flow and healing.

Rehabilitation and prevention
After the pain subsides it is important to regain flexibility and strength in the injured muscle. Gentle stretching will improve flexibility and help to avoid scar tissue formation. While the muscle is healing, working the surrounding muscles where tolerable may help to speed recovery by increasing blood flow and limiting scarring. Use of proper protective equipment during activities and avoiding impact to the thigh will help prevent thigh contusions.

Long-term prognosis and surgery
Proper treatment of a thigh contusion will ensure that there are no future complications. Flexibility and strength should return to normal after rehabilitation of the injured muscle.

Quadriceps Rupture

Classification: Acute

Brief outline of Injury

A *quadriceps rupture*, or strain, is a stretch or tear of the quadriceps muscles and/ or tendons. The quadriceps muscles are involved in supporting the structures of the hips and knees, and play a large role in supporting the weight of the body when standing. A quadriceps rupture can result from a forceful contraction of the quadriceps or it can be caused by unusual stress placed on the muscles. As with other strains it is graded 1 through 3, with 3 being the most severe tear.

The quadriceps muscle is actually composed of four separate muscles that work together to flex the hip and extend the knee. The four muscles of the quadriceps are the *rectus femoris, vastus lateralis, vastus intermedius*, and the *vastus medialis*. The most common place of rupture is where the muscles converge to form the quadriceps tendon, which connects to the patella, or knee cap.

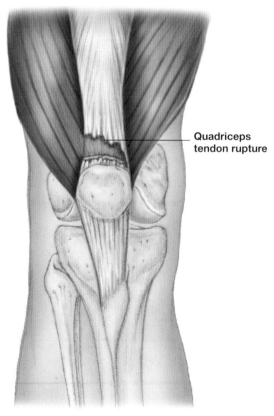

Quadriceps tendon rupture

Right leg (anterior view)

Cause of injury
Excessive overload of the quadriceps muscle. Forceful stretching of the muscle, especially during contraction.

Signs and symptoms
Pain and tenderness in the quadriceps, ranging from very little in a Grade 1 to debilitating in a Grade 3. Ability to walk may be affected, causing a limp or, in the worst case, a complete inability to bear weight. Swelling with Grades 2 and 3.

Complications if left unattended
Pain and tightness in the quadriceps will continue to get worse without treatment. The tightness in these muscles could lead to further knee problems. Grade 1 and Grade 2 strains left untreated can continue to progress to a Grade 3 rupture.

Immediate treatment
Grade 1: Ice, anti-inflammatory medications.
Grades 2 and 3: R.I.C.E.R., anti-inflammatory medications, seek medical help if a complete rupture is suspected or if unable to walk without aid. Heat and massage can be used after 72 hours to promote blood flow and healing.

Rehabilitation and prevention
Gentle stretching after the initial pain subsides will help speed recovery and prevent future recurrences. Strengthening the quadriceps is also important. When re-entering activity a proper warm-up must be stressed and a gradual increase in intensity should be followed.

Long-term prognosis and surgery
Quadriceps ruptures that are fully rehabilitated seldom leave any lingering effects. Complete ruptures may require surgery to repair and long-term rehabilitation.

Quadriceps Tendinitis

Classification: Chronic

Brief outline of injury

Quadriceps tendinitis, like other versions of tendinitis, involves inflammation of the tendon. Minor tears may also occur in the tendon when the stress is too much for the tendon to handle. This can be a result of repetitive stresses to the quadriceps, such as when accelerating and decelerating, or excessive stress before the muscle is conditioned to cope with it. Pain just above the kneecap, especially when extending the knee, usually accompanies this injury.

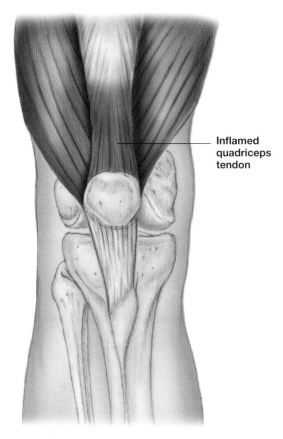

Inflamed quadriceps tendon

Right leg (anterior view)

Cause of injury

Repetitive stress to the tendon such as running, jumping, etc. Repetitive acceleration and deceleration as in hurdling or football. Untreated injury to the quadriceps.

Signs and symptoms

Pain just above the patella. Pain is aggravated by jumping, running, kneeling, or walking down stairs.

Complications if left unattended

The quadriceps muscles may also become inflamed, and the tendon will become weak if left untreated. This could lead to a rupture of the tendon. A change in gait or landing form can lead to other injuries as well.

Immediate treatment

Rest and ice. Anti-inflammatory medications.

Rehabilitation and prevention

Rehabilitation should include stretching and strengthening exercises for the quadriceps. Activities such as swimming can be helpful to reduce the stress on the tendon during this phase. Return to a normal activity schedule should be delayed until pain subsides completely and strength is restored. Keeping the quadriceps flexible and strong will help prevent this condition.

Long-term prognosis and surgery

A full recovery with no long-term disability or lingering effects can be expected in most cases of tendinitis. Surgery is only necessary in extremely rare cases of the condition.

Subluxing Kneecap (Patellar Dislocation)

Classification: Acute

Brief outline of injury

A *subluxation* is a partial dislocation of the kneecap, whereby the kneecap slides partially out of the groove in which it is designed to travel. Pain and swelling may accompany this condition. Athletes who suffer from a muscle imbalance or a structural deformity, such as a high kneecap, have a higher risk of a subluxing kneecap. This condition can also happen with forceful contractions, such as planting to change direction or landing from a jump.

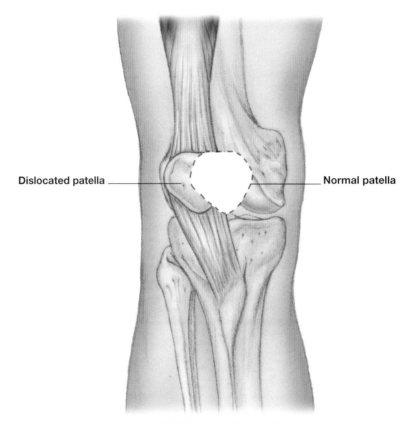

Dislocated patella — | — Normal patella

Right leg (anterior view)

Cause of injury
Strength imbalance between the outer quadriceps group and the inner quadriceps group. Impact to the side of the kneecap. Twisting of the knee.

Signs and symptoms
Feeling of pressure under the kneecap. Pain and swelling behind the kneecap. Pain when bending or straightening the knee.

Complications if left unattended
Continued subluxations can cause small fractures in the patella, cartilage tears, and stress to the tendons. Failure to treat a subluxation could lead to chronic subluxations.

Immediate treatment
R.I.C.E.R. Anti-inflammatory medications.

Rehabilitation and prevention
During rehabilitation, activities that do not aggravate the injury should be sought, such as swimming or cycling instead of running. Strengthening the vastus medialis and stretching the vastus lateralis will help correct the muscle imbalances that may cause this condition. A brace to hold the kneecap in place may be needed when initially returning to activity. To prevent subluxations it is important to keep the muscles surrounding the knee strong and flexible and avoid impact to the kneecap.

Long-term prognosis and surgery
Subluxations respond well to rest, rehabilitation, and anti-inflammatory measures. Rarely, surgery may be required to prevent recurring subluxations due to misalignment or loose support structures.

Tibiofibular Joint Dislocation

Classification: Acute

Brief outline of injury

The tibiofibular joint is the point where the tibia and fibula of the lower leg connect. This junction is at the inferior surface of the lateral epicondyle of the tibia, just below the knee joint. The tibiofibular joint only allows for very limited movement between the two bones. A *tibiofibular joint dislocation* is most commonly caused by a high impact injury, such as a fall onto a bent knee with the foot pointing inward (inverted).

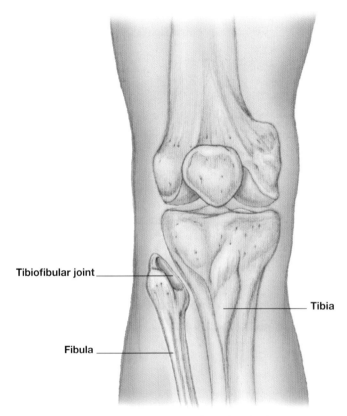

Tibiofibular joint

Tibia

Fibula

Right leg (anterior view)

Cause of injury
Impact to the knee or lower leg. Twisting of the knee.

Signs and symptoms
Pain and swelling around the lateral epicondyle. Pain on weight bearing. Pain when bending or straightening the knee or ankle. In some cases there is a visible deformity at the joint.

Complications if left unattended
Dislocation of the tibiofibular joint causes tearing of the ligaments that hold the joint together. This results in the knee joint being considerably more prone to successive dislocations and other injuries.

Immediate treatment
Rest, ice, and immobilization. Seek medical attention immediately.

Rehabilitation and prevention
During rehabilitation, activities that do not aggravate the injury should be sought, such as swimming or cycling instead of weight-bearing activities like running. Strengthening the muscles around the knee will help to provide support. A knee brace may also be used to provide extra support when initially returning to activity.

Long-term prognosis and surgery
For relatively minor dislocations a closed reduction is used where the bones are placed back in line using manual manipulation, which does not require any incision or opening of the joint. Where the dislocation is quite severe, surgery is usually required to fix or attach the bones back together.

Resources

Anderson, D.M. (chief lexicographer): 2003. *Dorland's Illustrated Medical Dictionary, 30th Edition.* Saunders, an imprint of Elsevier, Philadelphia, USA

Anderson, M.K. & Hall, S.J.: 1997. *Fundamentals of Sports Injury Management.* Williams & Wilkins, Baltimore, USA

Arnheim, D.D.: 1989. *Modern Principles of Athletic Training.* Times Mirror, MO, USA

Bahr, R. & Maehlum, S.: 2004. *Clinical Guide to Sports Injuries.* Human Kinetics, IL, USA

Beachle, T. & Earle, R.: 2008. *Essentials of Strength Training and Conditioning, 3rd Edition.* Human Kinetics, IL, USA

Delavier, F.: 2010. *Strength Training Anatomy, 3rd Edition.* Human Kinetics, IL, USA

Dornan, P. & Dunn, R.: 1988. *Sporting Injuries.* University of Queensland Press, Qld, Australia

Jarmey, C.: 2008. *The Concise Book of Muscles, 2nd Edition.* Lotus Publishing, Chichester, UK; North Atlantic Books, Berkeley, USA

Jarmey, C.: 2006. *The Concise Book of the Moving Body.* Lotus Publishing, Chichester, UK; North Atlantic Books, Berkeley, USA

Klossner, D.: 2006. *NCAA Sports Medicine Handbook.* The National Collegiate Athletic Association, IN, USA

Lamb, D.R.: 1984. *Physiology of Exercise.* Macmillan Publishing Co., NY, USA

Levy, A.M. & Fuerst, M.L.: 1993. *Sports Injury Handbook.* John Wiley & Sons, Inc., NY, USA

Martini, F. Timmons, M. Tallitsch, R.: 2008. *Human Anatomy, 6th Edition*. Pearson Benjamin Cummings, NY, USA

Micheli, L.J.: 1995. *Sports Medicine Bible*. HarperCollins Publishers, Inc., NY, USA

Meyers, T.: 2009. *Anatomy Trains, 2nd Edition*. Elsevier Limited, NY, USA

Norris, C.M.: 1998. *Sports Injuries: Diagnosis and Management*. Butterworth Heinemann, Oxford, UK

Reid, M.G.: 1994. *Sports Medicine Awareness Course*. Sports Medicine Australia, ACT, Australia

Rushall, B.S. & Pyke, F.S.: 1990. *Training for Sports and Fitness*. Macmillan Education Australia, NSW, Australia

Sports Medicine Australia: 1986. *The Sports Trainer*. Jacaranda Press, Qld, Australia

Tortora, G.J. & Anagnostakos, N.P.: 1990. *Principles of Anatomy and Physiology, 12th Edition*. Harper & Row, NY, USA

Walker, B.E.: 2011. *The Stretching Handbook, 3rd Edition*. The Stretching Institute, NY, USA

Walker, B.E.: 2011. *The Anatomy of Stretching, 2nd Edition*. Lotus Publishing, Chichester, UK; North Atlantic Books, Berkeley, USA

Glossary of Terms

Achilles tendinitis—Inflammation of the Achilles tendon.

Active stretching—Stretching exercises performed without any aid or assistance from an external force. This form of stretching involves using only the strength of the opposing muscles (antagonist) to generate a stretch within the target muscle group (agonist).

Acute injury—Injury from a specific event, leading to a sudden onset of symptoms.

Anterior tibial compartment syndrome—Rapid swelling, increased tension, and pain of the anterior tibial compartment of the leg. Usually a history of excessive exertion.

Arthropathy—Any joint disease.

Atrophy—A wasting away or deterioration of tissue due to disease, disuse, or malnutrition.

Articular dysfunction—Disturbance, impairment, or abnormality of a joint.

Avulsion fracture—Indirect fracture caused by compressive forces from direct trauma or excessive tensile forces.

Baker's cyst—Swelling behind the knee, caused by leakage of synovial fluid which has become enclosed in a sac of membrane.

Bursa—Fibrous sac membrane containing synovial fluid, typically found between tendons and bones. It acts to reduce friction during movement.

Bursitis—Inflammation of the bursa.

Capsulitis—Inflammation of a capsule, e.g. joint.

Chondral fracture—Fracture involving the articular cartilage at a joint.

Chondromalacia patellae—Degenerative condition in the articular cartilage of the patella caused by abnormal compression or shearing forces.

Chronic injury—Injury characterized by a slow, sustained development of symptoms that culminates in a painful inflammatory condition.

Collateral ligaments—Major ligaments that cross the medial and lateral aspects of the knee.

Compressive force—Axial loading that produces a squeezing effect on a structure.

Compartment syndrome—Condition in which increased intramuscular pressure impedes blood flow and function of tissues within that compartment.

Contracture—Adhesions occurring in an immobilized muscle, leading to a shortened contractile state.

Contraindication—A condition adversely affected by a specific action.

Contusion—Compression injury involving accumulation of blood and lymph within a muscle. Also known as a bruise.

Cruciate ligaments—Major ligaments that criss-cross the knee in the anteroposterior direction.

De Quervain's tenosynovitis—Inflammatory narrowing tenosynovitis of the abductor pollicis longus and extensor pollicis brevis tendons.

Dynamic stretching—Stretching exercises performed with movement.

Epiphyseal fracture—Injury to the growth plate of a long bone in children and adolescents; may lead to arrested bone growth.

Fasciitis—Inflammation of the fascia surrounding portions of a muscle.

Fracture—A disruption in the continuity of a bone.

Iliotibial band syndrome—Pain / inflammation of the iliotibial band, a non-elastic collagen cord stretching from the pelvis to below the knee. There are various biomechanical causes.

Inflammation—Pain, swelling, redness, heat, and loss of function that accompany musculoskeletal injuries.

Innvervation—Nerve supply to a body part.

Ischemia—Local anaemia due to decreased blood supply.

Larson-Johansson disease—Inflammation or partial avulsion of the apex of the patella due to traction forces.

Menisci—Fibrocartilagenous discs withinthe knee that reduce joint stress.

Meralgia paresthetica—Entrapment of the lateral femoral cutaneous nerve at the inguinal ligament, causing pain and numbness of the outer surface of the thigh in the region supplied by the nerve.

Metatarsalgia—Condition involving general discomfort around the metatarsal's heads.

Microtrauma—Injury to a small number of cells due to accumulative effects of repetitive forces.

Nonunion fracture—A fracture in which healing is delayed or fails to unite at all.

NSAID—Nonsteroidal anti-inflammatory drug.

Osgood-schlatter disease—Inflammation or partial avulsion of the tibial apophysis due to traction forces.

Osteitis—Inflammation of a bone, causing enlargement of the bone, tenderness, and a dull, aching pain.

Osteoarthritis—Noninflammatory degenerative joint disease, characterized by degeneration of the articular cartilage, hypertrophy of bone at the margins, and changes in the synovial membrane. Seen particularly in older persons.

Osteochondritis dissecans—Localized area of avascular necrosis resulting from complete or incomplete separation of joint cartilage and subchondral bone.

Overuse injury—Any injury caused by excessive, repetitive movement of the body part.

Paralysis—Partial or complete loss of the ability to move a body part.

Passive stretching—Stretching exercises performed with the aid of another person or apparatus.

Patellofemoral stress syndrome—Condition whereby the lateral retinaculum is tight or the vastus medialis oblique is weak, leading to lateral excursion and pressure on the lateral facet of the patella, causing a painful condition.

Plyometric training—Exercises that employ explosive movements to develop muscular power.

Posterior compartment syndrome—Pain in the posterior compartment of the lower leg, including soleus, gastrocnemius, tibialis posterior, flexor digitorum longus, and flexor hallucis longus. Site of pain varies depending on muscles affected.

Prognosis—Probable cause or progress of injury.

Propriceptors—Specialized deep sensory nerve cells in joints, ligaments, muscles, and tendons sensitive to stretch, tension, and pressure, which are responsible for position and movement.

Q-angle—Angle between the line of quadriceps force and the patellar tendon.

Referred pain—Pain felt in a region of the body other than where the source or actual cause of the pain is located.

Repetitive strain injury (RSI)—Refers to any overuse condition, such as strain, or tendonitis in any part of the body.

Rheumatoid arthritis—Autoimmune disease, in which the immune system attacks the body's own tissues. Causes inflammation of many parts of the body.

Sacroiliitis—Inflammation (arthritis) in the sacroiliac joint.

Sciatica—Compression of a spinal nerve due to a herniated disc, a muscle-related or facet joint disease, or compression between the two parts of the piriformis.

Scoliosis—Lateral rotational spinal curvature.

Seronegative spondyloarthropathy—A general term comprising a number of degenerative joint diseases having common features, e.g. synovitis of the peripheral joints.

Sesamoid bones—Short bones embedded in tendons; largest is the patella.

Sesamoiditis—Inflammation of the sesamoid bones of the first metatarsal.

Shear force—A force that acts parallel or tangent to a plane passing through an object.

Snapping hip syndrome—A snapping sensation either heard or felt during motion at the hip.

Spasm—Transitory muscle contractions.

Sprain—A rupture or tear of ligamentous tissue.

Static stretching—Stretching exercises performed without movement.

Strain— A rupture or tear of muscle or tendonous tissue.

Stress—The distribution of force within a body.

Stress (march) fracture—Hairline crack of a bone caused by excessive repetitive stress.

Synovitis—Inflammation of a synovial membrane, particularly a joint.

Tendinopathy—Disease of a tendon.

Tendinitis—Inflammation of a tendon. Also known as tendonitis.

Tenosynovitis—Inflammation of a tendon sheath.

Anatomical Directions

Abduction—A movement away from the midline (or to return from adduction).

Adduction—A movement toward the midline (or to return from abduction).

Anatomical position—The body is upright with the arms and hands turned forward.

Anterior—Towards the front of the body (as opposed to posterior).

Circumduction—Movement in which the distal end of a bone moves in a circle, while the proximal end remains stable.

Contralateral—On the opposite side.

Coronal plane—A vertical plane at right angles to the sagittal plane that divides the body into anterior and posterior portions.

Deep—Away from the surface (as opposed to superficial).

Depression—Movement of an elevated part of the body downwards to its original position.

Distal—Away from the point of origin of a structure (as opposed to proximal).

Dorsal—Relating to the back or posterior portion (as opposed to ventral).

Elevation—Movement of a part of the body upwards along the frontal plane.

Eversion—To turn the sole of the foot outward.

Extension—A movement at a joint resulting in separation of two ventral surfaces (as opposed to flexion).

Flexion—A movement at a joint resulting in approximation of two ventral surfaces (as opposed to extension).

Horizontal plane—A transverse plane at right angle to the long axis of the body.

Inferior—Below or furthest away from the head.

Inversion—To turn the sole of the foot inward.

Lateral—Located away from the midline (opposite to medial).

Medial—Situated close to or at the midline of the body or organ (opposite to lateral).

Median—Centrally located, situated in the middle of the body.

Opposition—A movement specific to the saddle joint of the thumb, that enables you to touch your thumb to the tips of the fingers of the same hand.

Palmar—Anterior surface of the hand.
Plantar—The sole of the foot.
Posterior—Relating to the back or the dorsal aspect of the body (opposite to anterior).
Pronation—To turn the palm of the hand down to face the floor, or away from the anatomical and foetal positions.
Prone—Position of the body in which the ventral surface faces down (as opposed to supine).
Protraction—Movement forwards in the transverse plane.
Proximal—Closer to the centre of the body or to the point of attachment of a limb.

Retraction—Movement backwards in the transverse plane.
Rotation—Move around a fixed axis.

Sagittal plane—A vertical plane extending in an antero-posterior direction dividing the body into right and left parts.
Superficial—On or near the surface (as opposed to deep).
Superior—Above or closest to the head.
Supination—To turn the palm of the hand up to face the ceiling, or toward the anatomical and foetal positions.
Supine—Position of the body in which the ventral surface faces up (as opposed to prone).

Ventral—Refers to the anterior part of the body (as opposed to dorsal).